The Dance of Your Core Healing

TRANSFORMING YOUR MIND, BODY, & SOUL IN THE NEW WORLD

Copyright © 2013 Angelika Maria Koch
Published by Medica Nova, LLC, Taos, NM, USA
www.medicanova.net. All rights reserved

No part of this book may be reproduced in any manner whatsoever without written permission of the author except in the case of quotations embodied in articles, literature, or reviews with authorship cited.

Editing and Production Services:
Heidi Connolly (www.harvardgirledits.com)
Cover Design: Karena Domenico (www.karenadomenico.com)
Photos: Karena Domenico
Photo Subject: Angelika Maria Koch
Printed: United States of America

The purpose of this book is to support the reader in his/her quest for spiritual and emotional growth as well as deep and lasting physical well-being. No information contained herein is intended to be a substitute for medical advice, nor does the author intend that any suggestions be used as a form of treatment for physical, medical, or mental issues without the advice of a conventional medical professional or licensed health practitioner. This information is not necessarily considered mainstream medicine. It is left to the discretion of and is the sole responsibility of the user of the information presented in this book to determine if procedures and therapy described are appropriate for that person or patient. The information should not be construed as a claim or representation that any procedure or product mentioned constitutes a specific cure, palliative, or ameliorative. This information is provided in good will for informational and educational purposes only. For protection of privacy, all names mentioned in this book have been changed.

Library of Congress Control Number: 2013913095
Perfect Bound ISBN 978-0-9888379-0-4 / eBook ISBN 978-0-9888379-1-1
(1) Holistic Health (2) Alternative Medicine (3) Healing (4) Homeopathy
(5) Nutrition–Health Aspects (6) Mental Health (7) Psychology (8) Spirituality

The Dance of Your Core Healing

Angelika Maria Koch
DNM LCH H.N.H.Ir

Medica Nova, LLC
New Mexico, USA

Testimonials

"I know Dr. Koch to be a tireless advocate for each patient's inner vitality to throw off the "morbid influence" that inhibits optimal health. That's a special way of saying that she serves each person's God-given ability to reverse that which causes pain and suffering, and to embrace the vitality that is the body's birthright. She is a knowledgeable, caring, and relentless advocate for the joy of health, and thus is an integral part of people's processes to restore their best level of health possible."

– Dr. Jack Tips, N.D. Ph.D. C.Hom. C.C.N.
Author of *The Pro-Vita! Plan for Optimal Nutrition*

"Dr. Koch is amazing in her ability and knowledge to address the symptoms of an illness, but she is also very adept at getting to the root of an ailment with a loving and penetrating method of verbal interaction. In the process the patient is often amazed to see and understand the interconnectedness of body, mind, spirit, and emotions. Dr. Koch links the physical with the emotional, the personal, and the transpersonal within, and in that way reaches so much more of a person as she touches and heals the Being in each individual. The old paradigm is based on fragmentation, separation, and dualism; it is an honor to be an integral part of this big change of consciousness to see us into the New World."

– Mathilde Freeman, Breath Work Therapist

"Have you ever asked yourself, in these days of pharmaceutical advertising with the long lists of abominable drug side effects, what might be a better alternative? Might there be a gentle and holistic option, for example, that would really work to recreate your total well-being?

I have experienced this guidance and its results as a patient of Dr. Angelika Maria Koch. I have used several of her recommendations with a positive outcome, and I hope you will agree with me that in these difficult times we must make the right choices for our bodies, our minds, and spirits."

– Madeleine Herrman, Author

Acknowledgments

With deep gratitude, I thank my two sons Frederick and Satya who unconditionally understand the magic of allowing me to be by encouraging the manifestation of the best of me.

My life-long lessons and clinical practice are deeply cherished, as I have been given the opportunity to work with my patients on their unfolding healing journeys. You are the ones who have shaped me into what I am today. With all my love, I thank you for dancing with me.

With reverence for all my teachers of the past and future who consistently inspire and support my personal evolutionary dance.

And lastly, a grateful bow to my body, my teacher and healer each and every day.

Much Love.

I dedicate this book to the New World

Contents

INTRODUCTION · 9

MY STORY · 19

Core Mind

THE MEANING OF HEALTH & DISEASE · 35

INVITING YOUR ILLNESS TO THE DANCE FLOOR · 45

THE SIGNATURE OF YOUR DANCE · 59

DANCING WITH YOUR CORE WOUND · 71

Core Body

TOXICITY DANCES THROUGH THE BODY · 89

THE ESSENTIALS FOR YOUR BODY TO MOVE · 111

THE NATURAL TIMING OF YOUR DANCE · 127

LACK OF ENERGY & CELLULAR INFLAMMATION BREAKS THE DANCE · 141

CLEANSING THE CELLS TO DANCE WILD & FREE · 169

Core Soul

THE MEANING OF THE SOUL · 199

THE AUTHENTIC DANCE BEYOND YOURSELF · 217

ENSOULED BODY DANCES WITH EMBODIED SOUL · 243

RADICAL DANCING IN A SOULFUL PLACE · 271

YOUR ETERNAL DANCE INSPIRES & TRANSFORMS THE WORLD · 285

REFERENCES · 313

Introduction

I would believe only in a God that knows how to dance.

—Friedrich Nietzsche

It is February 14th, Valentine's Day, and a perfect day to start writing this book, *The Dance of Your Core Healing*. It is a day filled with love and sweet moments that demonstrate how much we cherish the loved ones in our lives. Today, some will take their lovers to a romantic restaurant or surprise each other with a delicious meal. Some will exchange presents, flowers, or symbols that represent their love for each other. And some might take their beloveds to the dance floor to sway arm in arm to the rhythm of the music of the night. They might look into each other eyes knowing that, in this very moment, life is in its rightful place, that this moment allows them for a brief flicker in time to forget their small, or large, personal problems. The dance will be beautiful as the trust they have in each other reigns over the moment. There may be other couples on the dance floor or others watching from the sidelines, all enjoying the synchronistic steps of the couple in love.

Soon the music lifts our lovers to even greater heights as they dance through the night hours. The distinction between the dancing couple and the music becomes less and less noticeable as a merging of similar vibrations unifies them. As they enjoy their dance of love, the rhythm of their breaths, their movements, the place, the music, and the surrounding environment are all melting into one experience, one moment. Their inner and outer worlds are now dancing together.

Introduction

Imagine such a feeling within yourself, a feeling of total Oneness, and an experience of non-separation ... the final ending of any duality between yourself and the world. Imagine you are the one swaying with your lover to the beat of this exquisite dance. Even if there is no one else, no lover or partner with whom to dance, envision you are the dancer of your dance. It is only you, your body, and the dance.

Learning how to form a union with yourself through the tangible process of your own healing is the core message of this book. To move you through this process, I use the experience of the dance and the dancer. As these pages unfold, you will become your eternal dance as well as learn how to let the dance move through you. It is the thread of dance that provides the underlying theme and frequency to my message.

Many years ago, I gave birth to my second son on this day dedicated to love. Therefore, this day not only represents universal love to me, but the ultimate well of creativity in itself.

The Art of Healing is indeed a journey of birthing a creative process that deeply addresses the mental, emotional, physical, and spiritual aspects of our lives. Healing involves every part of us, every cell, every drop of our blood, and all our willingness to participate in this life-changing metamorphosis.

In the clinical practice of integrated and educational natural medicine for nearly 30 years, I have seen countless patients, from newborns to the very elderly, for both ailing physical symptoms and emotional upsets. Today I can confidently say that true healing requires a totally new paradigm if we want to understand medicine, whether allopathic, alternative, or anything in between. We have arrived at a point in human evolution that demands a new relationship and a very different approach to the practice of medicine itself.

We are living at a time when modern medicine presents us with overwhelming amounts of new scientific information and fresh evidence of its almost miraculous skills and powers. We are also aware, however, of the many debilitating side effects of allopathic drugs and treatments, which often solely focus only on the suppression of physical (or other) symptoms. More and more people are raising their voices ever more

Introduction

loudly, following their inner primal instincts in recognition that true medicine speaks a very different language altogether. And while it may be challenging to understand and express, this "new language" of the body is actually an ancient one that has existed for over thousands of years. Current medical procedures, on the other hand, are based on practicality, including the labeling and treating of presenting symptoms, and are lacking in humanity and soul.

Yet, even alternative medicine is showing its limitations in effectively treating the complex cases of our patients. Over the years, having treated symptoms from simple colds to chronic depleting diseases, I have come to the revelation that there might be one common denominator responsible for all individual diseases and their healing processes. I believe this common denominator, which may be initially intangible and something that expresses itself through us individually, occurs in each expression and manifestation of us all throughout humanity.

Our cellular structures and bodily functions, our mental abilities, our emotional make-up, and our spiritual communications have all been birthed from one primal realm, a place that is the very core of ourselves. Our individual relationship to this very core determines if we live a joyful and creative life or if we experience life as a victim with its presenting uncomfortable physical symptoms. We are the literal creators of our lives, in particular when it comes to our physical energy and vibrancy. To be ill or healthy, therefore, becomes an expression of how severed our connection is to source, our inner wholesomeness, and to our external world. True healing represents the unification of the self-created versus the belief that "you" and "I" are two different essences in polarity. It is when we accept ourselves that love, the neutral frequency, brings healing to this separation and hence to the healing of humanity.

***

This core of connectedness exists at the very deepest part of your inner wound, and is the door to your liberation and healing. And we are all part of this transformative journey throughout our lives. No one is excluded as each one of us walks this evolutionary path to find and ultimately heal ourselves.

Introduction

We have all heard about the Mind, Body, and Soul Connection, and we all understand that our physical symptoms are not separate events running parallel to our busy lives. We also know that the quality of our thoughts and emotions have a profound impact on the body and health. This book is not about a newly developed method for healing your symptoms or about reinventing the wheel of health and disease. But it does provide a new way to view this wheel of health in order to understand its true nature. With this information, it is my hope that you will be able to see your own wheels of vibrant and optimal health as they make the turn and head in the right direction.

This book does not give you new techniques in meditation and visualization. It does not provide medical guidelines for healing your ailing body; nor is it a manual in self-exploration. Rather, this book is about the interrelationship and interplay between the Mind, Body, and Soul, with their intricate communication channels and unlimited potentialities in creating the multifaceted jewel called "You." Supporting this creation is the ongoing magical theme of dancing with a chosen partner, dancing with yourself only, and dancing the ultimate dance with your soul.

This book is purposefully written in simple and accessible language, yet is filled with the 21st-century, cutting-edge science of homeopathy, systemic herbology, cellular biology, nutrition, detoxification protocols, and psychology.

This book is all about taking back responsibility for nurturing and caring for your body, as well as understanding its miraculous and eternal dance within you. In these pages I clearly explain, step by step, why so many of us become so ill in today's world and how we can shift that paradigm of illness to become the masters of healing ourselves. I welcome each of you to feel inspired to choose a completely new way of living.

You are a brilliant multifaceted jewel fully capable of assisting in your own healing.

Introduction

In my practice, MEDICA NOVA, I use therapeutic tools like in-depth classical homeopathy, systemic herbology, iridology, sclerology, advanced biofeedback, and functional tests supporting the patient's cellular protocols. This unique combination of clinically proven and ancient healing systems provides me with a clear understanding of the patient's core personality as well as his or her physical core imbalances. In this way, selected tailored treatment protocols can be established that result in effective and lasting amelioration of presenting ailments. Let's start with a closer look at the aforementioned modalities in order to understand the overall concept of my work and this idea of "core healing."

HOMEOPATHY

Homeopathy is a complete therapeutic system of medicine that aims to promote general health and thus reinforce the body's own natural healing capacity. With its countless scientific proven protocols, homeopathy is a proud beacon of one of the most effective deep-acting vibrational therapies. Homeopathy is used by over 500 million people worldwide and is the most practiced and applied healing system (next to allopathic medicine). It recognizes that all symptoms of ill health are expressions of disharmony within the whole person and that it is the patient who needs treatment, not the disease.

The founder of homeopathy, Samuel Christian Hahnemann (1755–1843), reasoned that there must be some kind of subtle energy within the body that responds to the minute stimulation of "remedies" and that enables the body to heal itself. He called this principle of energy "the vital force" of the body. In fact, this is the very force responsible for the continuous operation of the body by coordinating its defenses against all disease. Vital force is the energetic substance, independent of physical and chemical systems, that gives us life. It is also the energy that is absent at our death. This energy is affected by all our input—by everything we do. For example, a lifestyle that exposes us to ongoing stress, poor diet, a lack of exercise, as well as hereditary or environmental disturbances will eventually result in disease, which manifests in the form of symptoms. Every disease, no matter how its complex symptom-

Introduction

atic tapestry, is an outward manifestation of the vital force's attempt to elicit the imbalance within. This most creative intelligence, inherent in all of us, functions to heal its host to its highest potential.

Homeopathy is a therapeutic method that clinically applies the "law of similars" and uses medicinal substances in weak or infinitesimal doses. The principle of "like can cure like," the basis of all homeopathy, would state that any substance that can make you ill can also cure you, or that anything capable of producing symptoms of disease in a healthy person can cure those symptoms in a sick person.

For the homeopath, the true meaning of health is expressed in its ability to adapt easily to environmental changes on the mental, emotional, and physical level. Disease is an imbalance, which always affects the whole person; the underlying disease, the imbalance, always exists prior to the localization of symptoms and its clinical labels. Homeopathy is an effective science with no side effects, is not addictive, works on the dynamic plane, and is thorough—and thoroughly—holistic.

By taking responsibility for what happens to our bodies we can then start creating for ourselves the balance WE want in our lives, and we can start turning into our own feelings, or inner sense of what is wrong with us. By developing this positive approach toward creating a healthy life for ourselves we can move away from automatically taking a defensive position toward illness. —Miranda Castro, RSHom, Homeopath

IRIDOLOGY

The science of iridology is based on the analysis of one of the most complicated tissue structures in the whole body: the iris. The eye is a fabulous instrument! In addition to its remarkable ability to translate wavelengths of light into nerve impulses for vision, it registers and reflects the nerve impulses from all over the body into a pattern, which reveals specific stresses and conditions that affect a person's health. The eye is directly connected with the sympathetic nervous system and spinal cord. Thus the eye is in direct contact with the bio-energetic, biochemical, structural, and metabolic processes of the body via the nerves, blood vessels, muscle fibers, and lymph.

Introduction

A qualified practitioner can discern from the markings or signs in the iris the reflex condition of various organs and systems of the body. These markings represent a detailed picture of the integrity of the body with its constitutional strengths, areas of congestion or toxic accumulations, and inherent strengths and weaknesses. Nature has provided us with an invaluable insight into the vital status of the health of the body by transmitting this information to the eye.

Most of the presented diseases are of a chronic (long- standing) nature. Iridology gives an essential insight to the development of these chronic diseases or the diminishing of that disease or inflammation. It is this tissue change that takes place in the patient that makes iridology especially valuable. Iridology offers a unique perspective to the concept and practice of preventive medicine. It is difficult to alert a person to the health problems that his or her particular body will experience, using (only) orthodox methods of analysis and diagnosis. These methods rely upon the appearance of clinical symptoms. The iris, however, can indicate a problem in its earliest inception long before disease symptoms are present. With this information, a health program can be developed which is tailored to the specific needs of the client, thus preventing the manifestation of disease. —Bernhard Jensen D.C. Ph.D., Master of Iridology

SCLEROLOGY

The word *sclerology* means the study of the hard, firm outer coat of the eye, known as the white of the eye, or *sclera*.

More than the study of the white part of the eyes, sclerology is a method of interpreting the red lines, colorations, and markings in the sclera as they relate to the whole body health. The sclera is revealing of many forms of dis-ease (stresses, imbalances, energy blockages) wherever they originate by the characteristics of the red lines and markings that appear, disappear, and reappear in the sclera. The sclera will register an imbalanced body chemistry or deficiency in basic nutrition, structural misalignments, nerve affections, weakness in physiology, as well as stresses in the mental and emotional aspects. Sclerology is not a

Introduction

diagnostic tool but addresses the 'whole person science' and therefore serves as an invaluable tool. —Dr. Jack Tips, N.D. Ph.D. C. Hom, C.C.N.

SYSTEMIC FORMULAS: A NUTRITIONAL BREAKTHROUGH

In my practice, Medica Nova, LLC, I use several excellent natural supplements, some of which are worth mentioning here. SYSTEMIC FORMULAS, created by Dr. A. Stuart Wheelwright and his team, are designed to provide the nutritional building blocks essential for the support and rebuilding of specific bodily systems. Many professionals have found that these formulas are unsurpassed in supporting the body's natural abilities. It is no surprise that they therefore hold the lead position for supplements developed in the field of quantum physics and herbology. During my years in clinical practice, the brilliance of Dr. Wheelwright and the cutting-edge teachings of Dr. Jack Tips, a protégé of Dr. Wheelwright, have deeply influenced my approach and the resultant success of my practice.

DR. JACK TIPS

I was fortunate to study with Dr. Jack Tips, who not only became my mentor, but later, my colleague. Over the last 10 years, Dr. Tips' most innovative and state-of-the-art teachings have not only influenced my practice on a daily basis, but have also completely transformed my personal consciousness about core healing. Each of Dr. Tips' articles, newsletters, and lectures is the work of a master in terms of in-depth knowledge and the ability to transform 21st-century scientific research into an accessible language that benefits us all. From the basic building blocks of optimal nutrition to the most advanced cellular biology, today Dr. Tip's wisdom underlies the fundamental training of every healthcare practitioner as well as educational materials for patients welcoming the renewal of optimal health. Dr. Tips is the author of 16 books on nutritional healing and lectures around the world on natural health and healing.

Introduction

Working with such excellent tools and many teachers has shaped my current practice of integrated and educational medicine. As my skills in natural medicine expanded, I began synthesizing these various tools into a unique and innovative approach. Over time, I developed more and more of my own signature in treating my patients and creating their tailored protocols. Through today, I continue this exploration to deepen my knowledge and pursue the ever-unfolding newest scientific natural healing programs.

My patients teach me a lot, without a doubt, as well, and my work would not exist without them. Yet the most intimate, raw, and liberating experiences have been learned via my own ailing body. My body became and remains my personal teacher and healer every single day. In this book, you will get to know me quite intimately through my life story and my past belief systems. You will experience my discoveries in healing myself. Using my own story and those of my patients as illustrative tools, I willingly expose myself to you and the public quite openly, marking this book as a tangible symbol of my own path to healing. I do this because I have always believed that it is the wounded healer in us that is also ultimately our liberator.

So, here we are at the beginning of an exciting journey leading you to your Mind, Body, and Soul. May I invite you now to step with me onto the dance floor? The music has begun. We take position, we look into each other's eyes, and we acknowledge each other's presence.

Now ... let's dance.

The Grace to be a beginner is always the best prayer for an artist. The beginner's humility and openness leads to exploration. Exploration leads to accomplishment. All of it begins at the beginning, with the first small and scary step.

—Julia Cameron

My Story

> My aim is to assist you in the communication of your inherent creative intelligence to heal itself and bring forth your pure potentiality. In this way, each and every one of us contributes to a better health for humanity.
>
> —Angelika Maria Koch

I was born in the late fifties into a very conservative German family whose life was deeply affected and sculpted by surviving World War II. As I represented the first generation after the war, I also carried very different hopes and dreams about my unfolding future. Two families, my mother's and my biological father's, as well as the one from the second marriage of my mother to my stepfather, influenced my early years, as both environments displayed a very similar energetic coding regarding my upbringing. My parents' adapted survival mechanisms had shaped their thoughts and belief systems, coloring and influencing every part of their lives. Looking back, they both were exquisitely equipped and skilled in meeting challenging life situations in quite a grounded and very practical German manner. Their identity was influenced by the idea of an inbred diligence and work attitude that could only be compared to that of a boot camp. My mother rarely allowed herself a vacation or any "down time," and even weekends were filled with her dutiful tasks. Her life, filled with high morals, clear virtues, and an incredible willpower to survive anything life presented also made her a very successful businesswoman.

My Story

My family did not receive the day of my arrival into this world joyfully, as their expectation of welcoming a boy was crushed by my female presence. The already-chosen name of Peter now needed to be changed to Angelika. My sister, then already five years older, couldn't tolerate my very existence. In fact, her pathological jealousy culminated in several attempts to eradicate me from her life, which were luckily never realized.

Six years after my birth, I was presented with my parents' divorce, leaving me with the radical and abrupt separation from my father. From the day he left, I was not allowed to mention his name anymore, and told to stop thinking about him. My mother remarried almost instantly and my emotional wounds were either suppressed or denied as the new life took over. At that time, I suffered from a severe toxic bronchitis causing me to miss most of my school year. Forced to contain my grief and shock of losing my father, my body had immediately reacted with a long-standing illness affecting my lungs. In Chinese medicine, the lungs represent grief and emotional sorrow.

My upbringing was imbued with a pace and energy that radiated methodical practicality and the attitude of "getting things done." As both my parents worked in the city, numerous child-minders contributed their input to my early years. Each day, I commuted by train to my school, as we lived in the rural southern Bavarian countryside in a farming village of only 200 inhabitants.

Although we lived a financially comfortable life, my parents' emotional realms were never addressed. Emotions were not permitted to be felt, by them or their children. The deep inner wounds of having survived a war controlled by the Hitler regime, loss, sheer trauma, and post-traumatic stress had left them with ready-made survival skills, yet without any tools to meet and heal their inner tumultuous emotional worlds. Any emotional hurt or pain was immediately transformed into focusing on another project or dealt with simply by ignoring it, not by talking about it. I was told which clothes to wear and how to tie my hair. In their presence I was expected to act and feel according to their viewpoints. I was not allowed to be me! I was not allowed to play freely!

My Story

As we lived in the country, my friends and classmates could only be seen during school hours. My parents did not allow any friends in the house; therefore even friendships were very limited or never explored. At that time, to be free entailed punishment, abandonment, and consequences. My experience of life could be compared with living in exile, rather than embracing and exploring an unfolding youth. In some ways, exile is not a space. It does not incorporate an inner and outer home, nor does it give a sense of departure and arrival or a sense of belonging. It is a void, which can only be described as a nowhere-land, a space we might pass through, but do not want to stay.

I more or less learned how to live alone with myself, and the surrounding Nature, to which I deeply connected. Living an inner expansive and enriched life in stark contrast with my outer controlled world ultimately estranged me from my family unit. At seven years old, I officially separated myself emotionally from my parents, taking the conscious vow to live only another few years in their house, ironically called "home," until I reached the age where I would have the courage to leave.

We all know this common scenario of disconnected and dysfunctional families. Many of you can relate to your own story going back in your memories of your ancestors' upbringings and limited belief systems. There is no intention here to blame my parents about what they thought was right and appropriate in their lives at that time. Instead, I hope my story will serve you solely in understanding the unfolding mystery of healing the depth of your inner core and achieving your personal freedom.

I was a delicate girl, sensitive and acutely aware of my environment. As I spent most of my school years traveling by train, many hours of the day were filled with silence and non-verbal communication. Looking outside the windows of the railroad car day after day and watching the passing landscapes going by gave birth to my inner world. I pretty much knew by heart each section of the passing forests, the casting shadows of the open fields during the morning and afternoon hours, the cloud formations in the sky, the animals grazing along the railways, and the commuting passengers who entered and exited the train. I observed in detail how Nature unfolded in spring, blossomed in summer, contracted in the fall, and went to sleep in the winter with the changing seasons. It was a quiet world in which I learned to feel and know myself. During these years, I became a master in the art of observation by engaging in a committed and intimate life-long relationship with Nature itself.

At home, living in the country and away from my few friends and school life, I continued to live inside my self-created quiet world. By now, my ever-changing child-minders, some of them with little knowledge of the German language, were mostly responsible for keeping the household in order and providing me with set regular meals. We never established close bonds or any friendship. I more or less became a sort of chore, one more domestic task. My personal needs vanished deep inside me and could only be seen and expressed within that inner spiritual realm. I rarely asked for help or support, as this would have caused rejection, misunderstanding, or even danger.

Due to the lack of verbal communication, my afternoon hours were filled watching scenes in Nature, mostly from a window of our living room. This kind of "being with silence and observation" became familiar to me, as it was already my pastime during my daily train journeys to school. In my garden, I knew the birds, the sound of the swaying branches of the tall pine trees, the green and mossy smell of the forest ground, the rustling sound of the fallen leaves, the smell of the flowers, the color of the grass, and the tangible encompassing silence that shaped the afternoons. Soon, I started to draw and paint these still-life images. Canvases were filled with oil paints or charcoal, inspiring me to refine my already detailed observation skills. These paintings were embraced by my parents and openly displayed along the staircase walls. Surprisingly, my parents enjoyed my artistic gift, yet were not aware of the actual circumstances or reasons behind my creations.

During these many years of being with myself, I also enjoyed standing in front of the mirror watching my body swaying to the rhythm and sound of music. I loved to dance!

When my parents and sister returned from their work and school in the evening, the house was again filled with sounds and verbal communications. Suddenly, two very different worlds collided, like two rivers converging into a large riverbed.

My Story

I grew up very much alone, feeling and experiencing the world around me singly, rather than through engagement in communicative relationships. On the outside, I was a friendly and innocent girl, yet on the inside I was focused more and more on training myself in keen observation and in feeling out my environment, skills which were already influencing and shaping my courageous and sharply determined character that stood in obvious contrast to my exterior appearance. You could say that I trained myself to sense my environment more the way an animal might with all its refined sensory faculties. Even as a very young child, my days were filled with sitting in my sand pit playing with creepy crawlies and finding refuge in the form of a soft bed under a huge weeping willow tree whose green and golden branches cascaded toward the ground and sculpted the most wonderful tent and womb. This tree became my friend and my officially anointed substitute parent during the day.

Sometimes my parents took me to their festive and glamorous business meals or cultural events, which felt utterly distant from my quiet yet colorful world of Nature. Their aim was to introduce me to their world of cultured education and high society. Personally, I felt totally out of place, and from the time I got there hoped these events would soon come to a close. Bored and already trained in detailed observation of even the smallest movement in my surroundings, I began to take my inner world into these public events. My skill of observation turned into a passionate and entertaining game as I watched, with great interest, the gestures, faces, and behaviors exhibited by the invited guests. Listening for the meaning of the words spilling from their lips, I searched for a sign of their real core, their true Self. Could I see or find in them a similar Nature-like quiet world or the peaceful frequency that I knew so very well resided within myself?

To my amazement, I realized that superficial masks and defense mechanisms were only somewhat successful in hiding their inner selves, revealing a very different story. For the first time, I saw and felt the human separation from its very core and its own humanity. After these social events, I shared these insights with my parents. "So-and-so is an alcoholic," I'd say, or "So-and-so is having an affair with the woman he was sitting with at the table." These pronouncements naturally upset them no end, as they highly regarded these people as important business partners, perhaps even friends. Their dismissal and condemnation of a young girl's insights was immediate and palpable. Yet so often, after some time, my findings and "research" at these events were proven perfectly true, a fact which left my parents embarrassed and amazed at the same time.

Later on in life, I recognized my ability to see behind or through the human veil as a fundamental tool of my work as a healthcare practitioner. William Blake called it "double vision," or the power of seeing through the surface of things to what lies beneath.

❧

Those early years taught me well. I became my own individual, acutely aware of the natural moving rhythms of life itself. Nature taught me about a world without words, without negotiations, without ego, without dominance or control, and totally accepting of the "is-ness" of the present moment, which in itself is in a state of constant movement and change. This still and quiet inner world became my abiding truth. You could say I became an advocate of Nature, and a spokeswoman representing its voice.

My parents certainly had a difficult time with me, as by then they were listening to a very outspokenly brave little girl whose goal was to defend Nature in all its forms of existence. We seemed to speak two different languages. We tried to meet somewhere in the middle, but our attempts were mostly in vain. Often I felt misunderstood, as I am certain they did, too. To me, my parents' personal yet external upheavals, all centralized around their work, seemed so out of balance compared to Nature's ever-changing, yet very balanced healthy flow.

I remember one vivid encounter that connected me with the boundless and spacious quality of Nature specifically, an event that initiated me into the realm of "the beginning and the end" of it all, a place of nothingness and fullness at the same time.

My Story

On a rare sunny afternoon when I was three years old, my mother, sister, and I spent the afternoon at the nearby lake. Its shoreline had been extended by truckloads of sand in order to create usable beaches. It was a beautiful day and the shallow water invited me to play. I walked farther down the beach into the water. Then, suddenly the ground opened up and I was sucked under the water's surface by the loose quicksand. As I spiraled down toward the bottom of the lake, I could see the glazing shaft of sunlight above my head diminishing into a smaller and smaller sphere of light.

I was in awe of this new experience of silence. Its boundless space offered sheer freedom, peace, and utter stillness. I completely fell in love with this moment. I was fearless and free! It never occurred to me that I was losing consciousness or that I might be drowning. If this was the experience of death, then it was paradise to me. The sensation of losing my physical boundaries and floating silently through liquid space... of having an experience that could possibly evolve into one called death had suddenly elevated my consciousness to an awareness of the state of living. Spiraling down the tunnel of my known inner world, looking up at the dimming sunlight, my entire being was engulfed with a vibration, one that can only be compared to pure love.

Imbued with a sense of detachment from the existing world, yet fully immersed in peace and joy, this moment of almost crossing over into another world was undoubtedly my initiation into my chosen field of work.

In my perception, the process of dying, or of losing myself to something bigger than myself, had emerged as a wonderful and exciting endeavor. Later on, remembering my own near-death experience and how it had liberated me of my conditioned or imprinted fear of drowning, this pull to enter into the oceanic depths of a patient's psyche that waits for liberation via an inner shamanic process slowly but surely captivated my attention. It seems the sheer act of nearly crossing over into another world had taught me what I needed to know to help others. Most patients who intentionally want to heal, have to—and will—arrive at this place of crossing over, either by resolving their emotional blocks or through some form of letting go.

My Story

Back at the beach that day, as suddenly as the quicksand had dragged me under I was being pulled out of the water. The beach was filled with a frenzied panic, people screaming, my mother in hysterics, and everybody running around trying to take care of me. I honestly couldn't understand why all these people were "overreacting," as my experience had been both wondrous and without fear. I had come back from a place of paradise, a place of source itself, a place where I felt completely at home and comfortable. There was no need for panic or anxiety. Unfortunately, I was too young to verbally convey this utterly blissful state of having been sweetly cradled by the elements of Nature. Even now, as a mature adult, I attempt to recapture that incredible feeling of freedom by immersing my face in water at the end of each day.

Then came the teenage years, and life took on a very different energy field. It was now even harder to convey my self-taught essence of life to the outside world. My conservative parents desperately tried to control and limit my life with all the mental and emotional weapons at their disposal. The daily arguments became unbearable for both of us. The final climax came during one night of physical violence where I clearly realized it was time to leave this place I might once have called home. With the first train at sunrise, I left for the unknown a young woman of 17.

The familiar train with its rhythmic rumbling wagons, the blue fabric with tiny sprinkled purple dots that draped each seat, the fingerprints on the windows...they all welcomed me. I was comforted by the names and love poems carved by lovers or poorly behaved teenagers in the window frames, the day-old newspapers littering the seats and floor, the advertisements plastered in the corner of the walls where they met the ceiling of the train, and the so-well-known passing green landscapes. They made me feel utterly secure and warm, in the midst of this emotional and painful life-changing event.

I was undeterred. Bold, courageous, and strengthened by the courage and steadiness of Nature itself, trusting in its unwavering love and care for me, not even a violent experience could change my relationship to my inner world of truth. Having lived for so many years "by myself," I naturally became fiercely independent and skilled in taking care of my own emotional and physical needs. Conversely, I also shielded myself from all offers of outside help or what might have been valuable support. You could say I was stubborn!

It is interesting how authors Gary Goldschneider and Joost Elffers, in *The Secret Language of Birthdays,* describe those born on my birth date: "They have the courage to push beyond boundaries imposed by either society or Nature. Their will to overcome, to go one step further, to break out of limitation is marked. Once they have progressed to the limit others have reached, it only remains for them to push on."

My school life slowly but surely came to an end, as I was more concerned with surviving daily life than curriculum studies. Life was extremely challenging and, yet again, somewhere inside myself I deeply recognized that I was living with a force, an energy that ultimately feeds and enriches us all, and a frequency that was expressing Nature itself.

Physically, the difficulties of life took a toll on my health. My body soon began experiencing all sorts of physical pains, from back pain to chronic migraines, severe bronchitis and chest pain, abdominal and digestive ailments, abscesses, and soon-to-be post-surgical (in the aftermath of several surgeries), to the type of pain with "no known cause." Pain became my daily experience. Pain became a living entity in itself, a thing that lived inside me and interfered with my capacity to live my life. I often called it *The Pain*, as if that were its name, like a person.

As I got older, things did not improve. By now my body was literally riddled with physical pain. I treated it with natural protocols and sometimes succumbed to predictably drastic and cruel surgeries. Vital organs were removed in the hope of ameliorating this unbearable pain. To my amazement, even allopathic painkillers didn't help, and only managed to leave me in states of drowsiness and confusion. I experienced physical pain day and night and my sleep was often interrupted. Different kinds of pain, all very intense, spread through my body like a slow burning fire and had become the rulers of my existence. Over time, I got so frustrated with my body that there were times I wished I could leave this pain-riddled shell. I was not suicidal, but was becoming increasingly disconnected from this ailing body.

My Story

For years, I felt my life was ruled and controlled by these wrenching sensations, yet somehow an unwavering willpower kept pushing me on to manifest my dreams and visions.

As the years went by and the pain stayed, however, I became distinctly sensitive to the frequency of control. Anybody who displayed the slightest tendency to control me, to try to change my hard-established inner world, was unconsciously met with an instant physical reaction of muscular tightness and suppressed emotional anger. If I found myself in a tightly controlled situation, the same thing happened. Since external triggers were plentiful, I kept reacting from my self-instilled belief system to defend my truth or the way I related to the world. Of course by now the way I related was through the physical experience of being in pain. It goes without saying that at the time I was unable to see the beauty and potentiality of my pain-illness, which was only waiting to be released and healed.

Already fiercely independent, I became a single mother with two beautiful sons and created my own income source. Overall, I lived a very autonomous life. You might even say I became an Amazonian warrioress. I made sure that I avoided situations at all cost that tasted or even smelled of control, oppression, or lack of support. I lived in four foreign countries, including in an Indian ashram, all of which took me far away from the place of my origin.

The choice of my partners often resembled the raw and intense mirror of my inner unresolved wounds. Naturally, in my relationships I chose free-spirited and artistic men who I imagined would lovingly inspire the manifestation of the unlived, yet free and boundless part in me. As you can imagine, the outcome of such unions only added to my already embedded emotional trauma.

My defense mechanism, based on the belief system that I had to defend myself against all incoming potential dangerous opinions or ideas, expressed itself in controlling my personal environment, and sometimes my loved ones. I became a perfectionist and master builder of that environment. If something in the house required maintenance, it was fixed immediately, leaving no room or any possibility of being controlled by an object in need or by the need to ask for external help.

My Story

The terrain of my early years had shaped my belief systems and conditioned my behavior. The extreme and strange circumstances of my childhood years had hardened my perception of life; I focused on the need to cultivate my own mental and emotional resources, yet was deeply in need of external appreciation. As there was no one to rely on for that appreciation, I had to rely on myself. It was only a matter of time before this hardened shell of protection would crack. It was only a matter of time before the physical and emotional intensity of my pain would make sure I could no longer walk behind the veil of my self-inflicted delusions.

The blow, of course, had to come. One day it suddenly became clear that "my way or the highway" (I thought of it as "hard way") was an inefficient, ineffective adaptation. I needed to soften my approach. But how?

It came to me that the only way to live an authentic life would be to let the old one go. I could not go on in the same way, without deviating from my current values and mindset. I would have to leave that whole value system—the one that admittedly had worn me down—behind in order to be reborn. I would have to learn to do things I'd never done before: to have interconnections with people, to create partnerships, both personal and professional.

I would have to learn that in this lifetime, in order to embrace a body free of pain I would have to accept the fact that I didn't need to protect myself day in and day out, or prove that my way of doing things was the only way to survive the challenges that presented themselves. I knew this would require that I cultivate my ability to be receptive to other people's ideas and to truly support their spirits.

This would be the most difficult thing I had ever done.

✌

There is no need here for going on about how I continued my conventional efforts to meet my long-standing, chronic physical, mental, and emotional wounds with allopathic pain-reducing drugs, depleting surgeries and their additional side-effects, or numerous complementary/

natural medicinal treatments. That, after all, is not the purpose of this book. Nor is a description of my time in psychotherapy, which was certainly a temporary help, but still held no cure and could not shift my physical agony. Hence my search for its primal cause was on.

I pursued this search with a diligent perseverance as I was determined to find the instigator or at least the specific event that had caused "all this" to happen. There must have been something or somebody that had acted as the final trigger for the collapse of my body. But as my search to find and heal myself only led to more unanswered questions, I felt more and more lost. I could not stop wondering: Why wasn't I successful?

It was through my work as a health practitioner that the transformation from illness and pain to health finally began to occur.

Having access to so much new scientific information and medical developments, particularly in the field of natural and integrated medicine, gave me the ability—over time—to choreograph my own healing system. This system was drawn from many different sources and teachers. As I saw my patients improving through the use of this system, as I witnessed their deep transformative changes along with the amelioration of their symptoms, I too started to heal—from the inside.

Today, I can say with joy that I am healthier than I have ever been as I finally reconnected with and accept myself for who I AM. Ultimately, the breakthrough in healing my physical pain did not come solely through any one technique: the newest cleanse, the best vitamins and minerals, a change in consciousness (regarding my relationship to life and my environment), or the letting go of destructive partnerships. Instead, it was a slow, ongoing multifaceted process, which involved patience, diligence, and the true willingness to heal—along with those excellent natural supplementation and homeopathic remedies. The true lasting breakthrough came when I accepted and was willing to consciously experience the true nature of my distorted and splintered personality. It was this process that resulted in the final transformation of my limiting belief systems. As I liberated myself from one chain at a time, my physical pains started to disappear.

My Story

I now know that it is when we truly are willing to meet and face the need for our core's healing that we also begin to see how that healing will impact our immediate environment. Like a brilliant multifaceted diamond, our efforts are reflected on the surfaces around us. Family dynamics or the work environment might shift. Certainly your relationships with loved ones and friends will go through their own process of transformation. This is because you are an energetic being, a transmitter of ever-changing vibrational currents that stream through your thoughts and emotions and simultaneously affect the vibrational world around you. Your personal evolution is intimately interwoven with your closest environment, but also on a larger scale, with the planetary realm. As soon as your healing process is set in motion, your life cannot help but change in all its facets. In my case, four days after starting to write this book, my biological father passed away.

Your Individual Healing Becomes the Healing of the World!

Core Mind

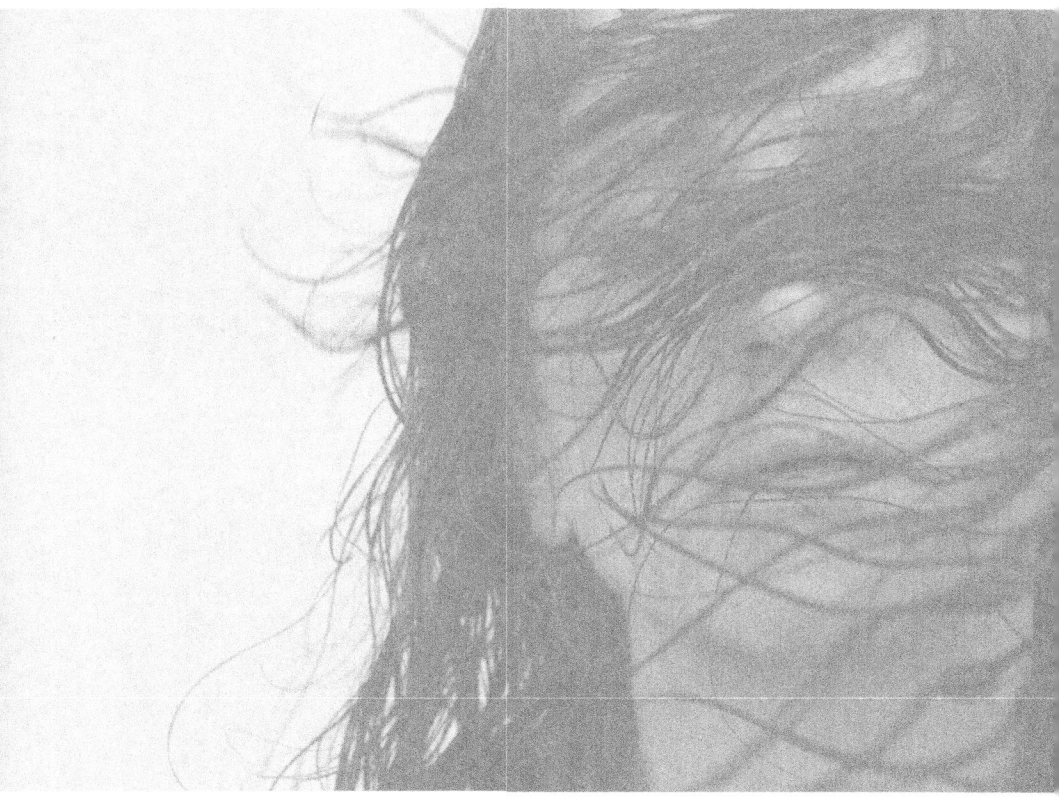

The wound is the place where the light enters you.

—Rumi

The Meaning of Health and Disease

> If someone wishes for good health, one must first ask oneself
> if he is ready to do away with the reasons for his illness.
> Only then is it possible to help him.
>
> —Hippocrates

Ask yourself this very simple question: What is the meaning of health? Today, we are easily satisfied with the idea that health simply means the absence of physical symptoms so we can function in our fast-paced and action-filled lives. But just because you do not suffer from your regular headaches or have recently had a break from your excruciating menstrual pain doesn't mean you are healthy overall. Far from it. If you accept this definition of health, you are depriving yourself of a whole new world, one that offers you the finest quality of life.

Optimal health is much more than the absence of disease. For holistic health practitioners, true health portrays itself in the ability to easily adapt to environmental changes on the mental, emotional, and physical level. This means you are not only free of physical discomfort, but also able to meet life's challenges with ease and the least amount of resistance. A truly healthy person radiates an inner and outer brightness, vitality, and an innate joy of life.

Health is much more than the absence of disease. It is a dynamic, vital, balanced, slightly ecstatic and aware state of being, which results from a relaxed and harmonious functioning of all the "bodies" or levels of the individual. —Dr. Jack Tips

Core Mind

Be honest with yourself. Does your life feel or look like Dr. Tips' description? Do you tap into your boundless source of creativity and optimal health on a daily basis? Does your body communicate with your core of vitality? Do you feel content inside yourself despite external global challenges like economic breakdowns, societal paradigm shifts, and environmental turbulence? Are you able to maintain a sense of self and soul in the midst of a crisis, such as having your house foreclosed on and seeing the sign on your lawn?

Today, our living conditions are far from perfect even if we choose to live in a relatively pristine, remote environment. Next to our genetic imprints, we all are affected by the ongoing environmental toxicity like carbon dioxide, agricultural and home-environmental pesticides, workplaces filled with chemicals, dry cleaning and hair salon chemicals, and air pollution from radioactive toxins to chemtrails. Our teeth are filled with silver amalgam dental fillings and we are exposed to countless x-rays procedures. Not to mention the onslaught of fast food containing growth hormones, preservatives, pesticides, and genetically engineered food articles. We expose ourselves with daily electromagnetic radiation from microwaves, electrical transformers, and personal cell phones, as well as geopathic stresses. From recreational drugs to the frequent use of antibiotics and prescription drugs to excessive alcohol consumption, we overload and stress our bodies day in and day out. Our children are bombarded with an onslaught of immunizations filled with mercury, aluminum, and formaldehyde, confusing their inherent immune systems and built-in defense mechanisms to disease. Today, none of us are immune or protected from any external toxicity. This huge adaptation causes stress for the mind and body. Our internal unresolved stories, intertwined with our external stresses, only leave us with a disoriented and torn inner tapestry. Today, no one is healthy anymore!

A totally new approach to the overall practice of allopathic and holistic medicine is therefore required. This approach needs proven, ever-deepening treatments that effectively emphasize the totality of our human existence on all levels, the mental, the emotional, and the physical.

The concept of treating the "whole person" is an essential element of holistic medicine. The basis of this belief is that symptoms, disease, and pain do not exist in isolation, but are a reflection of how the person as a whole is coping with stress. It is the whole person that counts—not just the physical body, but the mental and emotional bodies as well. If we truly want to embrace optimal health again, we are asked to look beyond the presenting complaint, beyond the label of the disease to the "totality of symptoms" the person experiences. Ever wondered when a child complains of an ongoing stomach pain that there might be a relationship to his parents' current divorce with their openly acted-out arguments? Or that the symptom the doctors are calling tachycardia (irregular heartbeat) might be forcing you to listen to your heart again, rather than listen only to your "logical" mind? Allopathic medicine exemplifies strong tendencies in specialization and in the reliance on analysis as the basic principle of its research, yet at the same time takes us further away from the picture of the patient as a whole.

For example, the commonly held belief in our society is that we are surrounded by antagonistic bacteria and viruses whose sole purpose is to attack human beings and cause them untold suffering. The allopathic approach is to remove these virulent organisms by creating a counterattack with antibiotics, anti-inflammatory drugs, and so on. However, germs and viruses in themselves do not only cause you to become ill, but are a secondary reaction in an already weak system of the body. Certain germs and viruses are actually part of the healing process, as they initiate sanitation of the affected area. If they are removed, the original acute disease may become more chronic or manifest as a more serious disease elsewhere in the body. We often confuse the cause of disease with the methods of recovery.

To graphically explain this concept, imagine a city during a week-long waste management strike struggling with millions of piled-up trash bags on its sidewalks and in its streets. Here, the appearance of the dreaded rats and flies is caused by the strike, which has caused the presence of the decomposing existence of the trash. The same principle can be seen unfolding within the body. The body is affected by illness due to a toxic inner terrain, and not only by the external stimuli that appear to cause the illness. If our immune system, the physical defense mechanism, our lifestyle, our relationship to life itself, and our connection to spirit is depleted and disconnected, we become susceptible to external stimuli like bacteria or viruses, which then resonate with our already weakened body.

It is therefore absolutely vital that all aspects of the ailing person are included in the treatment plan. Of course, this takes time, patience, respect, and a willingness to walk with the patient all the way to the very core of his or her healing journey. All medical practitioners of the healing arts, whether on the allopathic or the complementary side, should never forget that the well-being of the patient is the foremost aim. As times have dramatically shifted, today's skilled health practitioners have to educate themselves in many areas, from the anatomical and cellular functions of the body to the refined esoteric and psychological aspects of the human psyche. The profession of being in service to the well-being of humanity is intense and demanding, yet utterly rewarding for both the patient and the practitioner.

To be and live in a state of harmonious health we are asked to face our deepest shadows and unresolved wounds, as well as to dedicate a daily nutritional regime to our physical body in the form fresh organic food, excellent natural supplementation, daily exercise, and spiritual practices. To live in vibrant and optimal health requires daily attention to maintaining this wonderful state of being healthy. It is joyful work to ask for your willingness, dedication, and commitment, all vital ingredients in learning to dance with your life again.

༄

"Dis-ease" is therefore an imbalance that affects the whole person. First, one's vitality is affected, perhaps as a result of exposure to poor weather, lack of sleep, continuous stress, or a variety of other factors. When this imbalance persists, symptoms localize in specific areas such as the tonsils, neck, muscles, or stomach. In homeopathy, we refer to this localization as the *result* of the disease. The true disease, the *imbalance*, was there already, prior to the localization.

Disease manifests itself by signs or symptoms on the mental, emotional, and physical levels. It is a state of disharmony where the ability to adjust is lacking and the freedom to express one's creativity is limited. The presence and intensity of symptoms are therefore related to the body's ability or inability to adjust to changes to the environment.

In *The Healing Power of Illness*, Thorward Dethlefsen and Rüdiger Dahlke state: "Everything that happens within the body within any living being is the expression of a corresponding pattern, which is birthed deep from within his or her psyche and consciousness."

When you look at a spectacular painting that truly moves your heart, it is neither the canvas nor the paints that were used in the creation of such breathtaking masterpiece that has the effect, but solely the intention, the spirit, and consciousness of the painter himself that has transformed the otherwise invisible to become visible. Remember that every great book begins with a blank sheet of paper, just as every wonderful painting starts with an empty canvas. Every beautiful musical composition commences with a moment of silence. Every creative process, no matter how humble, requires you to bring forth something out of nothing. Using our example of the painting and the painter, we can see how the body then becomes a medium in the expression of messages that are initially purely manifested from thought processes and deeper levels of experience.

Applying this idea means understanding that the physical disturbance takes place initially within consciousness and is then transported into the body. If a person's relationship to life, his limited belief system, and his out-of-balance consciousness succumb into physical imbalance, we will then see this initially invisible force manifested into the visible form as symptoms. We are all too familiar with the unaware clinician who, after expressing his disrespect by stating, "It is all in your head! You are making this up!" leaves the patient stranded, angry, and confused, and in the role of a victim in relation to his ailing symptoms. The creation of a symptom goes far beyond the initial thinking process, something we will discuss further in the following chapters.

When disease presents itself, the body is communicating to us that our way of thinking, often unconscious, is out of harmony with what is beneficial to our being. Illness indicates the need for change in our belief system and tells us that we have reached our physical and psychological limits. Throughout life, we are taught that illness is bad and needs to be eradicated as quickly as possible. How about if we allow the possibility that illness is given to us as a gift whose purpose is to bring us back into equilibrium? The physical body does not create the dis-ease because the physical body can do nothing by itself. The body needs "you" to maintain its life, your soul, and your inner self. For example, instinctive reactions like the racing of the heart when we are nervous or the familiar butterfly sensation before a job interview are not coming from the body, but are transferred to the physical body through thoughts and emotions.

To be ill or to experience imbalances within the body is ultimately a reminder to love and reconnect with one's Self again. This goal certainly became the most important ingredient of my personal healing process. Even when unexpected and unpredictable events happen, we are still invited to see beyond the veil of the apparent meaning of these events. Nothing happens by coincidence! Nothing happens by chance! Your dance is already choreographed by your highest intelligence, which knows the time, the place, and appropriate moment to present you with the gift to your freedom. Disease is a human condition, which indicates that the individual is no longer in harmony at the level of his or her consciousness.

Referring to my personal story of multi-layered physical pain, I conducted a brief study regarding the following overall concept about the symptomatology of pain. *Time Magazine* (March 2011) published an article calling pain one of "life's most primitive mechanisms" by which even the simplest creature, if it has anything like a central nervous system, learns to avoid danger. Pain in itself is a protective sensation, the way the burning pain of your finger at a stove tells you to withdraw your hand. So, in essence, this sensation we seek most to avoid is in fact one of the most essential for our survival. But what happens when pain goes rogue—when instead of helping you get well or stay safe it becomes an illness in itself, as it did in my case? Then, we are talking about persistent and unceasing torment!

Time Magazine further educated us that 76.5 million Americans suffer from chronic pain (The Center of Health Statistics), with arthritis and back pain accounting for up to 60% of the cases. For much of the 19th and 20th centuries, opioids like morphine were the only weapons for stopping serious pain, with horrible side effects. Today, we overdose patients with acetaminophen, which in large doses causes equally serious health risks.

Chronic pain is one of the costliest health problems in the U.S., with an estimated annual price tag of close to $50 billion. Lower back pain is by far the most common complaint, affecting a staggering 70 to 85% of adults at some point in their lives and leaving about 7 million partially or severely disabled. Lower back pain accounts for 93 million workdays lost every year and consumes over $85 billion in health costs. Arthritic pain affects 40 million Americans, and 45 million suffer from chronic headaches. And people with chronic pain are twice as likely to suffer from depression and anxiety as those without. What starts in your lower back eventually eats away at your soul!

❧

I once wrote a story about Mr. Pain. Perhaps it will resonate with you, too.

Imagine you carry many heavy shopping bags, in fact way too many, and your body slowly starts telling you with its sore and aching muscles "This is all too much for me!" You realize you can't meet this task by yourself. To your amazement, Mr. Pain comes along and sees you struggling with your heavy load. Compassionately, he offers his help. He is willing to carry the extra bags and deliver them wherever you want them to go. You arrange with Mr. Pain that he will deliver your bags in the next few days. You immediately feel much better, really happy that somebody has come along to help you.

A short time passes, and you totally forget about the extra bags. One day, Mr. Pain comes to your home, rings the bell, and in a very friendly manner reminds you it's time to reclaim these extra bags. In fact, Mr. Pain explains to you that he has been carrying these bags now for quite some time and wouldn't mind lightening his load; in other words, he doesn't want to carry them anymore. And as Mr. Pain is a person with a kind, friendly, and caring nature, he really wants to make sure the bags are safely returned to their respective owner.

You look at Mr. Pain, totally amazed. Why is this person, apparently called Mr. Pain, suddenly at your doorstep asking you to take back some shopping bags? You can't remember ever meeting this person or that these shopping bags ever belonged to you.

Time moves on, and Mr. Pain gets increasingly impatient and angry. He keeps knocking at your door, shouting, screaming, and reminding you to take back the extra load you burdened him with in the first place. He reminds you of your responsibility to take back what is yours, all these bags that do not belong to him. At this point, however, all you want and need is space from this crazy person named Mr. Pain. By now, you will do anything to get rid of him, from prescribed pain-relieving prescriptions to pain-suppressive devices. But most of all, you feel very angry and depressed about Mr. Pain's presence in your life. "Why is Mr. Pain pestering me? Why is this guy in my life?" you ask.

The reality is that although Mr. Pain offered to carry your extra emotional baggage, the issues you could not face or solve at that time, he was expecting you would take it all back when the time came. For this is what happens in real life: at some point we are all asked to take back our own emotional baggage and face whatever it is in our life we have not dealt with or handled in the past.

Today, in the fields of psychology, metaphysics, and holistic medicine, we understand that every pain of our illness is the pain that was originally intended for somebody else, somebody who initially aggravated our life. Pain is always the result of some act of aggression. In my case, my suppressed anger and negativity was directed to anyone who literally or seemingly tried to control me or displayed a lack of appreciation. This blocked aggression turned into excruciating pain and became irrevocably intertwined with a multitude of physical symptoms. As pain or any illness is a vibrational force; it needs an outlet, like water freely running in its riverbed. If there is no exit valve, the blocked energy will target the weakest link within the system or the body to create a path for it to flow freely. The same principle is at work with our repressed emotions that ultimately start turning against us until illness appears as a general congestion within the body.

Health, on the other hand, displays free-flowing circulation on all three levels, the mental, emotional, and physical.

When a symptom manifests in the body it draws attention to itself, wanting to be seen and recognized, often seemingly interrupting our lives. The symptom, the pain, then becomes a signal, a pointer that directs our awareness to it and asks us to wake up, to remember the initial cause of the physical disturbance. Today, our language and choice of words regarding illness is in urgent need of change. We need to deviate from the notion that our bodies are "ill," when in fact only we, human beings, can be ill. Wouldn't it be inspiring for the physician to address the patient with the words, "Let's transmute your disease, and not fight it!"

Our human conditioning has us thinking and acting mostly with duality and self-division. For example, "He is more successful than I am," "She has more material possessions than I do," "He is more attractive than I am," or perhaps "She likes him more than she likes me." In the same way, we relate to disease and its presenting symptoms as separate from our existence, as if there is something "out there," something outside of us that we must "fix." We experience conflict due to our split consciousness that operates in opposites and in a primal separation from the whole. As we choose to participate in a fast-living world, we do not appreciate being interrupted or being taken away from our busy lives, and we do anything to eliminate that which interferes with our goals, especially when it comes to pain.

❧

We all bear witness in observing the intense yet natural process of polarization in the two-year-old child who identifies with himself by saying *No!* to almost everything in its presented world. We call this time period "the terrible two's," yet for the child its defiant negativity serves to solidity the growing personal self. By saying No! the child feels his identity and becomes the person with his chosen given name. We are taught to measure and compare ourselves to our external world. We are also asked, once grown up, to break through these once so eagerly cultivated conditioned boundaries. We live in a world reigned by a dualistic consciousness, and disease stands as a product of our own mental duality.

Healing, then, is the act of transcending our inbred cellular-polarity thinking. We can see this phenomenon even within our cell structures, an event which we call cancer today. Cancer is an expression of cells that have decided to separate themselves from the larger cell community and use that community as their host for the benefit of the individual's survival.

In *The Healing Power of Illness*, Thorwald Dethlefsen and Rüdiger Dahlke write: "It is illness that ultimately makes us Heal-able. Illness is the turning point, at which polarization can start to be turned into wholeness. But in order for this to happen, we have to lower our guard and instead learn to hear and see what illness has to tell us. We have to start listening to our inner selves and enter into communication with our symptoms if we are to learn what they have to tell us."

&

As soon as we separate from the whole-ness, mentally, emotionally, or physically, dis-ease is invited to the dance floor. And you are the one who will now choose its dance partner, called "physical discomfort." It is time to take your partner onto the dance floor by committing to your unfolding sweet liberation. The choice of your partner is perfect.... It is your dance!

As soon as you trust yourself you will know how to live.

—Goethe

Inviting Your Illness to the Dance Floor

> Only to the extent that we expose ourselves over and over to
> annihilation can that which is indestructible in us be found.
>
> —Pema Chödrön

By now you can see, and perhaps feel, that health and illness are complex realms that can only exist and be nurtured via our consciousness relationship to life, whether positive or negative. Today, either through the lens of allopathic or complementary medicine, we often blame solely external sources, like the germ, the bacteria, environmental pollution, or the internal heavy metal toxicity for our weak constitutional makeup. Of course, all these aspects play a significant role in physical tissue breakdown, yet should not be blamed as the prime cause of today's degenerative diseases.

The germ, for example, has been blamed long enough. It is time to boldly move forward into the 21st century with a better understanding of health, as well as to address the individual susceptibility to illness as the underlying cause of disease rather than continue to entertain the worn-out germ theory. Despite a relatively high standard of living for most of the population, including access to better nutrition, education and improved medical procedures, in regards to our health and well-being we still haven't really moved far from the overall conditions of less affluent nations of the world. Ask yourself the fundamental questions: *Why are our children not living their optimal health or glowing with vitality and intelligence? Why does one in every three people die of cancer in our society today? And why, over the last 40 years, have we been faced with diseases like chronic fatigue, fibromyalgia, candida, and AIDS despite all our medical advancements?*

One of my teachers once shared this insight: To stimulate a dormant disease into its manifestation or form, the body requires three primal ingredients. The first aspect entails the inherited history of the person and his physical weaker links. The second aspect addresses an unexpected event, like a trauma, which deeply affects the person's inner and outer world, and is curiously necessary for the inherited pool of dormant symptoms to be stirred up. Neither of these ingredients are the final deciding factors in the manifestation of the patient's latent symptoms, however. It is the third factor that will eventually make or break this situation. It is the patient's mental and emotional relationship to the traumatic event itself that makes the difference.

Let's have a look at an eye-opening example of past and current global wars occurring around our planet. Countless people have died unnecessarily and are still dying; countless people are still being tortured and raped. Many men, women, and children endure hardship beyond endurance, as well as the loss of their loved ones and families. There are some who express and experience war as the most difficult time in their lives, yet, as soon as the war officially comes to a close, they decide to move on despite their deep emotional wounds and scars. They start a new life! Then, there are some who will barely or never recover from their traumas and who find it almost impossible to even contemplate starting a new life again. It is the very relationship to their experienced circumstances that ultimately will be the deciding factor of any manifested future diseases.

We often sigh and feel relieved once a war is declared as "over," yet for most of the population who have experienced its horror, the inner war of their emotional and physical body has just begun. Psychotherapy or counseling sessions, designed for grief, trauma, and PTSD are immensely beneficial here, but limited in terms of the true core healing of the patient's physical imbalances. The inflicted person may mentally understand the connection between his body and ailing symptoms, and may feel his emotional wounding, but at this point his cellular transformation often remains untouched.

Each and every day, we are faced with presenting circumstances that only reflect our behaviors and actions in relation to our inner core wounds. In fact, we become and live our core wounds by projecting them onto our external world, both in relationships with people and with the environment in which we live.

C. G. Jung, imminent Swiss psychologist, described the sum of all the rejected aspects of reality that we cannot or will not see within ourselves, and of which we are therefore unconscious, as "the shadow." This thing called the shadow becomes our greatest threat. I choose to call this aspect within us our *core wound* as it lives within our unconscious realm and operates from the depth of our inner ocean, the place where we rarely want to go. Anything that the personal self rejects, criticizes, and does not want to approve originates within our core wound.

Today, our common understanding of medicine is still based on the English naturalist Charles Darwin's theory, which states that individual traits are passed through the generations. Darwin suggests that hereditary factors are passed from grandparent to parent and to child and control the characteristics of the individual's life. For decades, the medical establishment—and the rest of us!—believed that inherited physical weak links and genes controlled our lives, aside from all the external stimuli.

Bruce H. Lipton, Ph.D., highly acclaimed biologist, clearly enlightens us in *The Biology of Belief,* demonstrating that this belief system cannot sustain itself anymore, as genes cannot turn themselves on or off and are not self-emergent. Something in the environment has to instigate or trigger the gene activity patterns, either in the form of environmental influences, stress, including depleting nutrition, thoughts, or emotions.

The law of vibration says that everything in the universe is in a constant state of vibration. That is, everything, whether solid, liquid, or gas, is made up of energy, and all these forms are constantly moving and vibrating. A rock, your car, or you, a human being, constantly vibrates at the subatomic level. When we speak of *resonance*, we are expressing the concept that we can come in contact with things or people that have that same vibratory frequency, the same resonance that resides within us and with which we resonate. In other words, we feel in resonance with something or somebody if we recognize his, her, or its similar frequency and expression. This connection makes us feel comfortable, content, understood. On the contrary, if we are not aware and conscious of our inner core's wounds, we attract external circumstances and/or people who reflect (mirror) back to us this very unresolved frequency.

As author David Icke wrote in *Vibration Creates Matter*, "Your thoughts are a form of energy with their own unique frequency and as your thoughts are sent out into the universe they gather energy vibrating at the identical frequency and bring to you circumstances and people who reside on the same frequency."

Since we are generally unconscious about this fact, we easily feel emotionally reactive, particularly around challenging events or someone who has seemingly harshly affected our life. In this context, all organisms, including humans, communicate and read their environment by evaluating energy fields.

This sensing of energy fields reflects the same experience that I so often felt as a child. Watching the fleeting landscapes as I silently sat on my train and sensed each of its "containers of life," I knew that such experiences were my initial teachers, birthing in me the awareness of my own existence. Here, the invisible touched the visible, as well as my as yet invisible future life. Nature revealed to me its interconnectedness and its relationship to everything on this planet and beyond as expressed in its continuous rhythm and movements. Neither nature nor we are ever stationary or fixed, but part of the ever-evolving process called life. Our relationship to our immediate environment ultimately sets the stage for our future health as our thinking processes, both positive and negative, have a direct influence on our cellular structures and life span.

Using excessive recreational or prescription drugs is one way to suppress and silence the body's symptoms to such a degree that we are able to ignore our personal involvement with those symptoms. It is not my first choice to impress with numerical statistics, but we should be aware that iatrogenic illness, or the kind of illness induced by the adverse effects of prescribed medications, is the leading cause of death in the U.S. today and responsible for more than 300,000 deaths a year. This raw and brutal approach in meeting disease with ignorance and with an attitude reflecting the pursuit of personal power denies the presence of the ailment's energetic field and its transformative potentiality.

Today, we also know that almost every major illness can be linked to chronic stress. We are aware of the connections and links between our psyche and body, yet as practitioners still haven't found a clear and effective system for accessing the patient's overall emotional and mental state relative to his presenting symptoms of degenerative disease. We specialize in this and that field rather than develop a unified medical arena in which each and every approach is targeted and ultimately centralized to address the complete core healing of the patient. If we understood that the presenting symptoms of our diseases are the manifestation of the unresolved unconscious realm within ourselves, we would be eager to create a total different paradigm of medicine today, and would then relate to the term *symptoms* in a very different manner. Our cells do not control the body as its authority and master: it is the brain and the heart that influences the behavior and functions of our cells via the nervous system. Our inherent belief systems regarding everything we experience in life ultimately shape and form our mental, emotional, and physical health.

❧

Let's have a look at one of my patients whom I recently treated for high blood pressure. The gentleman, 55 years of age, had developed bouts of very high blood pressure over the last two years. He had also experienced an increase of ongoing family challenges, as well as some confrontations at work. He described his major symptom as being "unable to breathe," a sensation which was inhibiting him from following his weekly exercise regime. As this man was a sports coach for high-school teenagers, he was very concerned about whether he would be able to maintain his current profession. After collecting the initial appropriate facts of his symptoms and family history, I asked "B. M." to tell me more about himself, something that described him more clearly. B. M. immediately replied, "I am not so good with conflict, particularly in situations where harsh words are expressed. I really don't want to deal with these current family disputes. Personally, I am really guarded about raising my voice. I am a calm person and do not want to get involved in these conflicts."

When I asked B. M. to describe the emotional experience of the high blood pressure attacks, he answered numerous times in the same way: "I feel anxious, really anxious, and very tense." He then continued to describe how he felt the same anxious feeling when he had to face any conflict, either within the family or at work. His words were, "Here we go again . . . it's like a loop, and I can't get out of it!"

First, let me explain something about high blood pressure and its metaphysical meaning, so you can relate to my patient's chosen words describing his symptoms and his life in general.

Blood represents the river of life! Without it, we would literally dry up and die. Blood nourishes us with essential nutrients and acts as a life-bringing transport system for all of our organs. Blood "pressure" symbolizes the interplay of fluidity and free-flow versus the resistance of the blood vessel walls. As blood represents the individual's vitality, so does its resistance or limitation ultimately mirror the resistance to external barriers in life. Blood pressure can rise with excessive activity, but can also rise by simply thinking about any unpleasant situation. Today, through experimental research, we know that one's blood pressure can go up if the conversation gets too close to a person's particular conflict theme, but soon goes down again when the individual starts talking consciously about his present conflict. If the person diverts his accumulated energy blocks by constantly thinking about a certain unresolved issue, however, without undertaking any physical activity as an outlet for his elevated blood pressure, he actually creates an ongoing pressure within himself.

My patient's attitude about avoiding any conflicted situations along with his self-inflicted anxiety-ridden inner pressure was stimulating his cardiovascular system, which was normally primed to engage in physical activity or some sports regime. When this type of outlet of energy release did not happen, he began living under the strain of the huge pressure rising from within. My patient's inability and sheer refusal to meet and face conflicts in his life had resulted in the direct expression and manifestation of high blood pressure. His relationship to conflict was passive and non-engaging in nature, as he generally avoided it altogether. He didn't want to be dragged into this "loop," as he so eloquently called it. Yet by avoiding the loop of his struggles, he was unconsciously inciting a non-flowing loop in his own blood. My patient was more or less looking from the outside in at his conflict, rather than finding the necessary resolutions within his life. And, as he was not looking at the excessive internal pressure as a sign that he needed to resolve his conflicts, his physical blood pressure kept going up.

People who experience high blood pressure often have a tendency to divert this excess pressure into physical activity like sports. My patient had been an athlete, but had been forced to slow down his activities by becoming a sports coach for teenagers.

Individuals with high blood pressure carry a lot of frustrated aggression relative to facing major conflicts in themselves and with other people who they perceive are causing these conflicts. My patient restrained himself from facing his uncomfortable family and work situation, therefore adding to the constriction of his blood vessels while his suppressed aggression about the conflict raised his blood pressure. In reality, this patient's emotional experience is in direct relationship to his symptomatology.

Once we understand that each and every physical expression has its mental and emotional counterpart we can carefully choose the most appropriate vibrational treatments and remedies that are capable of dealing with the totality of the person, rather than trying to heal the individual parts. Homeopathy is such a vibrational medicine, able to address this delicate subject of meeting the whole-ness of the person. I will explain homeopathy's beauty and efficiency more in the coming chapters.

High blood pressure can also become a predisposing factor for heart attack. In this case, repressed anger becomes manifested in a more blocked aggressive energy and then released in a heart attack, meaning the heart literally tears apart or the person gets "stroked." If my patient hadn't chosen a natural and effective treatment that included the deep healing of his emotional inner wound, his initial high blood pressure condition could have resulted in a heart attack, which would have been a sure indication of the totality of all the previous emotional attacks that my patient had failed to resolve in the past.

The concept of mind-body connection is more than familiar to us today, yet when it comes to actual situations we often seem to forget this vital interconnection. The manifestation of disease is inspired and activated within us by the inbred polarization of our conscious and subconscious mind. As we live an inner and outer duality, so does our body in relation to its life-giving source and us.

Bruce Lipton describes the subconscious realm like this: "Our subconscious mind is like an emotionless database of stored programs whose function is strictly concerned with reading environmental signals and engaging in hardwired behavioral programs, no question asked, no judgment made. The subconscious mind is similar to a programmable hard drive into which our life experiences are downloaded. When an external stimulus is perceived, via the nervous system, it will automatically engage the behavioral response that was learned when the signal was first experienced." In other words, our subconscious mind is like an autopilot that reacts to any environmental disturbances. Its nature can be compared to a genie in a bottle, which obeys and acts according to your commands, whatever they are, good or bad.

Now we can understand why our cell's behavior doesn't cause the actual disease, as the disease is created by an instilled behavior based on an inflicted belief system received via the nervous system and the brain that eventually influences the cell's behavior. Furthermore, these subconscious behaviors might not even be part of our own nature, as they are often learned programs stored internally by watching other people, like the family and community members with whom we grew up. This is the reason our children, who have copied us from an early age, repeat these learned behaviors into their adult years and then pass those same behaviors to their children.

Core Mind

How you think, feel, and act determines your physical biology. Ask yourself: *What are my beliefs? What are my expectations? What are my habits, desires, and fears? Which kind of relationship influences me the most? What is the quality of my surrounding environment? Is it life-affirming or hostile?*

Your life choices have a direct link and consequence to your hereditary blueprint and the genes within your body. As soon as you change your life to go in the most positive direction, your cellular behavior and overall life span is instantly affected.

I will briefly explain this phenomenon by taking a deeper look within the body and the cells, as this same concept applies within the body as without.

❧

In today's scientific community, the newest and most spoken-about field is called *epigenetics*. *Time Magazine*, in the article "Why Your DNA Isn't Your Destiny" (Jan. 2012), states: "At its most basic, epigenetics is the study of changes in gene activity that do not involve alterations to the genetic code but is still passed down to at least one successive generation. The cellular material, called the epigenome, governs these patterns of gene expression. It is these epigenetic marks that tell your genes to switch on or off, to speak loudly or whisper (health or disease). It is through epigenetic marks that environmental factors like diet, stress and prenatal nutrition can make an imprint on genes that is passed from one generation to the next."

Each and every strand of your DNA is wrapped, or encased, by a "sleeve" of complex proteins called *epigenes*. Your genetic blueprint will always be the same as it was at birth, but the behavior of your blueprint can and will change according to specific external triggers. With the intentional input of your positive thinking processes, your epigenes can tell your DNA to prevent the growth or the amelioration of a tumor or the onset of a degenerative disease. This switching on and off of a gene is called *methylation*, and our knowledge of this "switch" truly holds hope for healing and for the future of new medicine. It all boils down to your created environment of thoughts, feelings, and behavioral reactions, which directly influence your healthy or diseased body. Your epigenes are sculpted by your experiences. Remember, the incoming information from your surrounding environment, as well as your mental and emotional input, are as critical as your internal environment, as they influence who you are. Your environment affects your genes, your health, and well-being.

This new exciting emerging science of epigenetics literally means "controlling the genes from above" (due to the patterns of gene expression that are governed by the cellular material—the epigenome—that sits on the top the genome) focuses on the fact that our cellular expression is ultimately influenced and regulated by our external realm of experiences, rather than our internal world called DNA. And this mind-blowing process all happens in your cell membranes, the true brains within your body. As the world, or external environment, affects your thoughts and emotions, your thoughts and emotions equally affect your cellular behavior. As above; so below…and as the macrocosm is reflected in the microcosm, and vice versa. We will talk more about the wonders of epigenetics in *Core Body*.

The subconscious mind is larger and much faster than the conscious mind, and can account for as much as 90 to 95% of the mind's overall activity each day. Our lives are shaped not by who we are, but how we learn to be! With 60,000 thoughts a day and an overall high percentage of negativity in its content, the body is literally bombarded with negative imprints. Today, our life is a printout of our subconscious minds. Our thoughts and feelings are converted into chemicals that affect the function of the entire body and well-being. Feelings of hopelessness, helplessness, or worthlessness, just to mention a few of the more difficult emotions, are subconsciously formed belief systems that are intrinsic to our destiny. This subconscious and on-going program does not recognize time. It is experienced in the present tense, as if its reaction were being experienced for the very first time, although each reaction has really happened in the recent past. This is the reason we often confuse reality with delusion, as our behavioral experience feels so real, so very present. But remember, what we learn from our family, culture, or community does not define who we are in our core Self.

You have heard these words before, but they apply here more than ever: You cannot solve the problem by repeating the same thing that created it! You have to step outside your thinking into a space of conscious awareness in order to see the true creator of your belief system. You have to become present about what *is*.

Gregg Braden, author of *The Spontaneous Healing of Belief,* says: "Belief is the program that creates patterns in reality. Many of our most deeply held beliefs are subconscious and begin when our brain state allows us to absorb the ideas of others before the age of seven. When our soul hurts, our pain is transmitted into the body as the spiritual quality of the life force that we feed into each cell."

Our instilled beliefs act like colored glasses in front of our eyes. You believe what you see and see what you believe! Our inherent biology is intimately intertwined with our beliefs and therefore cannot be separated from our healing process. Your disease or presenting symptoms are the window to your liberation, and only by dancing with them together, and doing it with joy and love, will you be able to embrace your complete healing.

Healing is made possible only by making ourselves aware of those hidden aspects of ourselves that are our shadow and by integrating them. Once we have discovered what we are lacking, the symptoms become superfluous. —Thorwald Dethlefson and Rüdiger Dahlke

Through the cultivation of clear self-consciousness we can override learned behavioral programs with a renewed sense of self-empowerment and freedom of choice. You are not the victim of your disease, as your body isn't the enemy threatening you. As soon as your mindset changes, the biology of your body changes automatically. Your positive and negative beliefs impact every part of your life and result in vibrant and optimal health or decay. As soon as we take our attention from and lose awareness of our conscious mind, subconscious behaviors can take over, leaving us stranded as victims of a body in pain. As mentioned earlier, any causal therapy can highlight the situation with mental and even emotional understanding, yet is limited in its ability to achieve the final breakthrough of our cellular energy fields. This complete resolution can only be achieved when we dare to go a step further, a step that will lead us deeply into the experience of the belief system itself.

Deepak Chopra, in *Reinventing the Body, Resurrecting the Soul*, writes: "Trust begins by recognizing the signature of each emotion. Each one is a sign that you are resisting. An experience is creating stress, and that happens because instead of flowing through you, that experience has hit a barrier. May be you can't see what's going on, but your body can feel it. Feeling is the first step of tearing down barriers and no longer needing them."

In my personal story, true healing wasn't found in the realization of multiple causes, such as the annihilation of my female presence at birth, the sudden interruption of my mother's breast milk, my unusual early solitary upbringing, the mental and emotional control mechanisms of my parents, or even the pathological jealousy of my sister, but only though the awareness of my reactions and relationship toward the totality of all these experienced circumstances. The true cause of all these years of multiple physical pains was, and still is, to be solely found within myself and not in the projection of specific or fractional pieces within the whole story. The mind and ego may be satisfied by such an assessment temporarily, but our behavioral reactions will continue to affect our overall physical symptoms.

My physical body was reacting to the totality of my immediate environment in proportion to my conflicted soul. Remember, the environment affects our cellular behavior, not only the incoming bacteria or virus. It is the overall energetic field in which we live that determines our cellular and human behavior. My personal story served my evolution well in order for me to heal aspects within myself that could only have been addressed via this perfect mirror of choreographed circumstances. Every symptom we experience offers us both a challenge and an opportunity. Once we understand this phenomenon, that illness actually serves us to heal and find ourselves, we start to relate to its symptomatology with a softer and sweeter heart. Your illness is the window to your freedom!

Core Mind

Let's not forget . . . we are still dancing on the dance floor. The current song comes to its end and a new one is about to begin. The rhythm and tone is different, and for a brief moment you and your partner re-align yourselves with its new frequency. You take in the first few notes, listen acutely to it play; you may even feel compelled to close your eyes to feel its flavor. Then, the moment comes when you and your partner feel comfortable enough to fall and let go into the music, both deciding to engage in this new dance. Having had already the opportunity to dance together, you now feel more at ease with each other. Each dance feels lighter and more effortless as you and your partner are daring a bit more in the repertoire of each other's steps. By now, you even develop your own signature of your dance. Let us explore this unique expression: your "signature," or how you feel and manifest physical symptoms within your body.

If you begin to understand what you are without trying to change it then, what you are undergoes a transformation.

—Jiddu Krishnamurti

The Signature of Your Dance

One day your heart will take you to your lover. One day your soul will carry you to the Beloved. Don't get lost in your pain, know that one day your pain will become your cure.

—Rumi

You are invited to a party and all your friends will be there. As you enter through the front gate of your friend's house, your ears are filled with all sorts of noises, from people laughing to the glasses clinking to the beat of the music. The party is in full swing and everybody is having a great time. The music blares from the speakers and the dance floor is packed with dancers dancing to the rhythm of the sound. As your eyes scan the dance floor, you can't help looking at one particular person who stands out of the crowd. His arms fly freely around his body, swirling in synchronistic rhythm to the base and percussion beats of the song. You find yourself magnetized by his courage and freedom in letting himself fall and merge with the music, seemingly unaware of the other people around him. His movements are not learned or choreographed, but pour effortlessly from his body. His body dances with grace and in unison with its untouchable source of existence. As you keep watching his "being in movement," you also feel inspired and somehow stimulated in daring to feel your next dance within your own freedom.

Core Mind

The dancer's dance has become his signature, the expression of its individual frequency. His dance is unique and cannot be duplicated. It belongs only to him.

Physical illness, in its expression of chosen symptoms, is also unique only to you, not to anybody else. If ten people are affected with a common cold, each and every one of these ten people will express unique symptoms solely relevant to their individual presentation of that cold or flu. Allopathic prescribing is based on the "law of contraries," which advocates that an illness should be treated by a substance capable of producing opposite symptoms in a healthy person. For example, common diarrhea is treated with aluminum hydroxide, which produces constipation. The person might experience temporarily relief, yet the initial symptom of diarrhea has also been simultaneously suppressed and deadened in its energetic frequency. The symptom of diarrhea was there for a reason, trying to communicate with its host regarding a physical imbalance in need. Due to the allopathic prescription, the person's innate communication with his body was disrupted.

Homeopathy always works on the law of similars that we discussed earlier. A frequency-like remedy is chosen, one that resonates with the frequency of the person's personality, his symptomatology, and his life experience. It all matches up, like the dancer above who became his dance. Homeopathic remedies act as catalysts, meaning the remedy stimulates the body's own vital force, or immune system, to heal itself. The homeopathic remedy acts like the music or the song that stimulates the dancer to create the most dynamic and harmonious dance fueled solely by his individual source of creativity.

The concept of signatures was first introduced by Paracelus (1493–1541), the "prince of physicians," who contributed much to the understanding of the "doctrine of signatures." Today, this phenomenon can still be seen, especially in the plant kingdom, where the color, shape, or part of a plant indicates its use in the cure of ailments and where each characteristic of the plant has some relationship with the presenting physical complaint. During Paracelus' time, it was thought that this stamp, or signature, was placed on the plant by a guardian angel! For example, plants with yellow flowers or roots with yellow sap can treat jaundice, a condition where the eyes and face take on a yellowish tint. Red-colored roots can treat bleeding symptoms, as they resemble the color of the blood. If you ever watched poplar leaves, which belong to the aspen trees, shaking in the summer breeze, you've noticed that these leaves shimmer in a peculiar way. Known to us as "quaking aspen leaves," they resemble a similar quaking movement that we see in the symptomatology of Bell's Palsy. This doctrine of signatures is still subscribed to by herbalists today and certainly stands as a nonverbal, informative, and medicinal transmission among many indigenous tribes.

In Paracelsus' own words: "The proposition is that signatures in form denote a resource, compatibility, and affinity between certain minerals and gemstones, plants with herbs and flowers, animals, and Man, out of which conclusions may be drawn about the sources of Man's stress and disorders, especially those of mind and emotion. So the form and the essence are one thing."

Again, the dancer becomes his or her dance. In my early twenties, for nearly seven years, I lived in an ashram in India. I was a disciple of Bhagwan Shree Rajneesh, later called Osho. At the end of each day, we all gathered in a large, elegant, roof-covered open space called the Buddha Hall where hundreds of sannyasins (disciples of Osho) danced their own unique dances fueled by an energizing live band and sweetly embraced by the golden setting sun. These dances became my closure of each day, a living and dynamic meditation.

Once Bhagwan said to me, "Angelika, when you dance, dance with all that you have inside yourself as this might be your last dance!" I never forgot these words, and even today I remind my patients to wholeheartedly embrace and welcome their healing journeys with all they have inside themselves.

Everyone, especially someone afflicted with illness, speaks in a psychosomatic language that clearly speaks of his inner truth. Literally all his chosen words and hand gestures are signals of his symptom's energy field and magically refer to his physical experiences and identified belief systems. Often, the person conveys his entire mental, emotional, and physical conflict within 10 minutes of the first consultation. He unconsciously chooses words or sentences that portray the frequency and the hidden revolving door to his deep and transformative healing. We live the total experience and sensation of our illness through our body and, in reverse, our body communicates back to us the expressions of all our psychological conditions and processes.

Our language includes many speech idioms that we unconsciously use to describe our emotional situations. After a painful divorce or separation, for example, we might speak of a "broken heart" or, when describing a truly wonderful moment in life, we might refer to "my heart leapt for joy." When a situation seeks emotional expression we might say "It feels like my heart is bursting with emotion," or that "I feel something heavy in my heart." A sensitive person might describe herself as "taking everything to heart" or as being "softhearted." We speak of people who are "half-hearted" and others who are living their lives with an "open heart." And what about the person who tells his lover that she is "close to his heart"?

A skilled physician listens with a refined ear to these colorful verbal expressions as they represent the key to the temple of renewed optimal health. Symptoms force us to make changes in our lives, either through our behaviors relative to the illness itself or in the form of a complete external change, like a residential move, a new job, or a change in our relationships. On one hand, they can stop us from doing what we initially intended to do; on the other, they can force our hand to make us do things we never intended to do in the first place. Your illness will change you and your resistance to it will ultimately only hinder your evolutionary progress, which is guided by your soul whose only desire is to embrace you as a whole again.

Your recent ski accident might have been an unconscious way to give yourself a much-needed break, or your broken leg might be an indication that you are consciously or unconsciously suppressing violent thoughts directed at someone else. Your debilitating asthma attacks, the ones where it's easy to inhale but exhaling occurs with great difficulty and results in the experience of suffocation, might signal that you take on too much and are having problems delivering. If your head is stuffed up and your nose blocked due to congestion from, could it reflect the emotional situation with your boss, about which you keep saying, "I have had it up to here!" while drawing a line at the height of your nose? An upset wife complaining about her marriage and her re-occurring urinary tract infections with burning urine may be reflecting the emotional state of her suppressed anger and her feeling of being "pissed off" in general. The person with burning and cramping stomach pains and a recent sudden job loss might say, "I feel as if I was punched in my stomach." Someone with a sore throat and complaining of an unbearable situation at home might express it in this way: "I just can't swallow it anymore," again portraying a clear ongoing relationship between the mind and the body.

Best-selling author, Louise Hay, was one of first recognized authorities who illuminated us all with her book *You Can Heal Your Life* (Hay House, 1984) in which she explains how our beliefs and ideas about ourselves are often the cause of our emotional problems and physical illness and how, by using certain tools, we can change our thinking and our lives for the better. Her books continue to affect millions who learn how to manifest truly desired lives, including more wellness in their bodies, minds, and spirits.

M. T. is an 18-year-old young woman of mixed race who suffers from an unpleasant psoriasis on her legs and arms. Her self-consciousness regarding the unsightly red skin patches reminds her each and every day of something she needs to hide from the external world. She often feels ashamed, and somehow "ugly." Being of mixed race and living a less than wealthy lifestyle, she experiences equal shame and a need to hide these facts from her friends and peers, while compensating for this inner conflict by being an overachiever. The very physical symptom of the psoriasis that makes her more noticeable compels her to negate herself, to hide herself and her personal life from the outside world. The conflict is devastating to her.

Physical symptoms are not solely related to mentally or emotionally created belief systems. In this case, the patient's itchy skin was also aggravated by a gluten sensitivity and other food allergies. Yet, to simply prescribe a topical medication like a corticosteroid cream for the itchy and flaky skin would clearly be nothing more than a temporary Band-

Aid, assisting only in pushing the psoriasis further into the patient's interior where it would slowly begin to affect the next organ in line, the lungs. The core healing of this teenager would have to include the totality of her physical symptoms and mental belief systems in order to establish any or lasting amelioration.

R. D., a 44-year-old male, suffers from chronic digestive problems. R. D. contacted me because he had already seen multiple gastrointestinal specialists as well as alternative practitioners. He was desperate, as nothing seemed to help. He reports that his stomach feels bubbly and that he gets easily bloated, a condition accompanied by lots of flatulence. In his daily life, R. D. also displays obsessive behavioral patterns regarding his food intake. He makes sure he eats at particular times only; if he can't eat at that given time he becomes extremely anxious. If he hasn't had his set meal in the evening he eats during the night, just to make sure he won't starve. He describes his situation like this: "If I feel restricted in getting a certain amount of food in I have to make up for it. I get really anxious if there isn't enough food in the house. I feel like I am starving and I can't miss out on any meal. If I wake up during the night and don't eat, I feel exhausted because I'm now thinking, how much do I have to eat to make up for the missing hours I haven't eaten? It is a daily survival in relationship to food."

R. D. started to experience his first anxiety attacks during puberty. He lived with his mother and was strangely, singularly focused on her presence. Sometimes, when he slept overnight at a friend's place, he woke up terrified and questioning, "How am I going to live by myself when I am older? How am I going to support myself when I leave my home?" He felt totally overwhelmed whenever he stayed away from his mother or his home. Today, any stressful situation, either at work or in relationships, feels distinctly like these past events.

In this example, we can really see that R. D.'s digestive symptoms can only be healed if his mental belief system about how difficult it would be to survive if he were away from his mother, the point of nurturing, and later about his relationship to food, are deeply explored and understood.

Core Mind

F. G., a 58-year-old male, was diagnosed with digestive imbalances and high blood pressure. He has recently suffered a stroke with a narrowed right coronary artery and major restriction of his left artery. Over the last five years, he has experienced intense family stress dealing with his divorce and his inability to communicate with his daughter on a regular basis. Ongoing verbal fights have caused him to experience a whole spectrum of emotions. He describes himself with the following words: "I always run and hide to places where others can't get me. I always have escape routes! I am careful and I get worried if people see my inner stuff, me being vulnerable. Then they can control me and then they can affect me. I am not like a solid structure, I am more like an eggshell, and I get hurt easily."

F. G.'s verbal expression speaks of an inability to face conflict, an energetic pattern very much related to high blood pressure.

F. G.'s situation intensified when his daughter decided to break off any contact with him. The patient often felt that his daughter was carrying her parents' unresolved issues and equally living in emotional pain. In his words: "I am aching as my daughter is suffering and I can't stop her pain. I am on the outskirts and I have to accept that she has to go through that. I want to be a good guy, and it hurts me that my daughter thinks badly of me. My relationship is now screwed up with her and I've lost her. I feel like I am hanging off the cliff and the rope is frail. If I make the last wrong move, the rope will break. So I can't make a mistake now. I felt totally crushed when my daughter told me she didn't want to talk to me anymore."

Again, the avoidance of conflicting situations can cause heart problems. In this case, the deep emotional heartbreak caused my patient the inevitable stroke to his brain and lack of circulation to his heart. His heart was as broken as his "inner rope," which finally gave way by narrowing his arteries.

After the stroke, F. G. wrote to me: "What I am beginning to understand about myself is that I am obviously a very stressed person and this has caused the excess secretion of adrenaline, which affects the arteries by eventually hardening them." Here, too, in order to save F. G.'s brain, heart, and arteries from further incidences not only was an effective natural supplement program indicated, but also a therapeutic vibrational tool like homeopathy to heal his broken heart and mend his habitual escape pattern from challenging conflicts.

E. C., a 60-year-old female, presented to me after having recently returned from a family vacation on a cruise ship to Europe and suffering from extreme vertigo and dizziness. As she can't bend down or move quickly without feeling instantly dizzy, she has had to interrupt her work as a teacher. Initially, she didn't want to participate in the cruise as several family members were invited, including her brother's wife with whom she struggles to get along. For the first two days on the boat, E. C. experienced seasickness because the weather was stormy and the sea was rough. She describes the journey as a crushing disappointment as the constant tension with the family members was affecting her deeply. In her own words: "It felt like the ocean waves were inside me! I felt anger, resentment, and depression . . . and I am all holding on to it. I feel off-balance!" When I asked her to describe the actual experience of being dizzy even though she's back on land, she responded, "I feel like I am still on the ocean hanging over a railing. I can't bend forward or look downward because immediately I feel like fainting." Initially, E. C.'s medical doctor prescribed anti-anxiety medication, which caused the additional side effects of more dizziness without any amelioration.

We can clearly see the relationship of mind and body in this case, too, where E. C.'s internalized and suppressed emotional upsets are manifesting in her symptomatology of feeling dizzy. Traveling on a large moving ship while experiencing a difficult family dispute had made her experience emotional vertigo.

A. S., a 54-year-old woman has been diagnosed with multiple sclerosis-like symptoms that include a staggering gait and spinal nerve affectations. By the time she comes to see me, she has had every possible medical intervention from the allopathic to the alternative. Her last spinal/cervical thermal findings indicated a pinched nerve and artery located between the upper back and neck due to spastic muscles that were affecting the nerves over the back of the head to the forehead. She was having esophageal irritation and improper digestion due to spastic function of the pyloric valve (the valve at the end of her stomach). A. S.'s gallbladder was also affected, as the valve between her small to large intestines was also spastic, or overly contracted. A. S.'s thoracolumbar fascia, the membrane covering the deep muscles of the back of the trunk, and spinal displacement had resulted in excessive stress to the exit of all affected nerve roots, all due to the overly contracted muscles. This woman was clearly ill!

Over the last few years, A. S. had been deeply affected by an ongoing and unresolved marital crisis. When I asked her to describe her life, she answered, "I am caught in the middle, between my husband and my children. I love him, but by now my children hate him. My neck, shoulders, and shoulder blades feel as if somebody's jammed my head into my spine. I feel totally disconnected! I keep up a shield to protect my children from any emotional pain, and I also have to keep up a shield to my husband in order to protect me from him."

I asked her to describe this idea of holding up a shield in more detail. "I feel as if I'm standing in a hallway. On one hand, there is my husband, and I put out my right arm to keep him away. On the other side are my children, and I put out the other arm to keep my husband away from them, trying to protect my children from him. This is taking all my strength! It is like I'm pushing these two heavy weights that are now closing in on me. I am bearing the pressure and I'm afraid I'll collapse."

Imagine standing in a hallway for just 15 minutes with both of your arms stretched out horizontally and pushing equally in both directions into an imaginary wall. I know that personally, even after five minutes, I would be shaking and trembling and possibly experiencing excruciating muscle pain streaming throughout my body. Perhaps my neck would seize up as well. This constant contracted and spastic emotional state, the inner life of this patient, was being directly reflected in the physical spasticity and nerve sensitivity in her body.

It would be irresponsible as a physician not to include this woman's life story into any treatment plan. Therapies like psychotherapy or counseling might be helpful, but not deep enough to facilitate cellular transformation. Here, too, we need to go a step deeper by applying an innovative and holistic approach to transform such deep and engrained belief systems.

Core Mind

In all these case examples, it is the body that lives and expresses its real story, the story that the patient must ultimately explore in his or her healing. We can see how our accumulated mental, emotional, and/or physical toxins correspond to the repressed conflicts within the psyche. Yet, ultimately, nor our thoughts, circumstances, or cellular toxins are to blame as the prime/primal cause of our illness.

Every symptom offers us a challenge as well as an opportunity to heal. If we choose to ignore the presence of our symptoms we not only prolong our physical crisis, but also stimulate the intensity of the ailment. The overall pain becomes stronger, the rash spreads to other parts of the body, and the initial irritable bowel syndrome now takes on the status of an ulcerative colitis.

My own physical pains were expressed in stabbing, cramping, burning sensations were of a mostly inflammatory nature, clearly reflecting my mental, emotional, inner, and outer inflammatory war as I attempted to protect myself by being in control. As I learned to push hard against any incoming, seemingly hostile frequencies, I applied the same principle to an equal degree to alleviating my intestinal pains by pushing hard against my body with my fingers or fist. This action often temporarily relieved the pain, yet clearly depicted the same frequency of my mental belief system, which was based on pushing through or beyond any difficult challenge in my life with the acquired survival skills of my past. My physical symptoms mirrored my limited and life-depleting belief system. Conversely, if a situation presented itself where I could not push through even after working at it, I got ill.

We tend to experience in life what we identify as within our beliefs. Only by finding the stillness in both polarities, the physical symptom, and the created belief system are we able to find true transformative freedom from all of it. When you open to the chaos of darkness within you, you will invoke—and evoke—the mystery of your life.

*

At this point in our journey, the common psychosomatic approach we've been discussing—that is, how to understand the mind and its direct link to physical symptoms—is indeed helpful and often results in the desired relief of ailments. Yet, ultimately, such an approach still only scratches the surface of any deeper healing. The initial understanding of the mind-body connection can create wonderful breakthroughs in our lives and capably lead us away from inflicted and stagnated life circumstances or physical discomfort, yet only marks our initiation to go further into the richness and depth of our personal evolution and the final merging with the soul. In the next and following chapters, you are given the opportunity to realize that deep and lasting wellness requires a completely new approach in meeting illness today.

Are you ready to go deeper?

It's time for another dance. The night is still young, and you and your dance partner decide to move to a more adventurous location. You both want to see the stars and feel the cooling breeze of the night. You open the doors to the back garden leading to an expansive porch, and with a leap of joy in your heart, you continue your dance under the luminous night sky. Are you ready now to give your all and dance all the way? Let's do it!

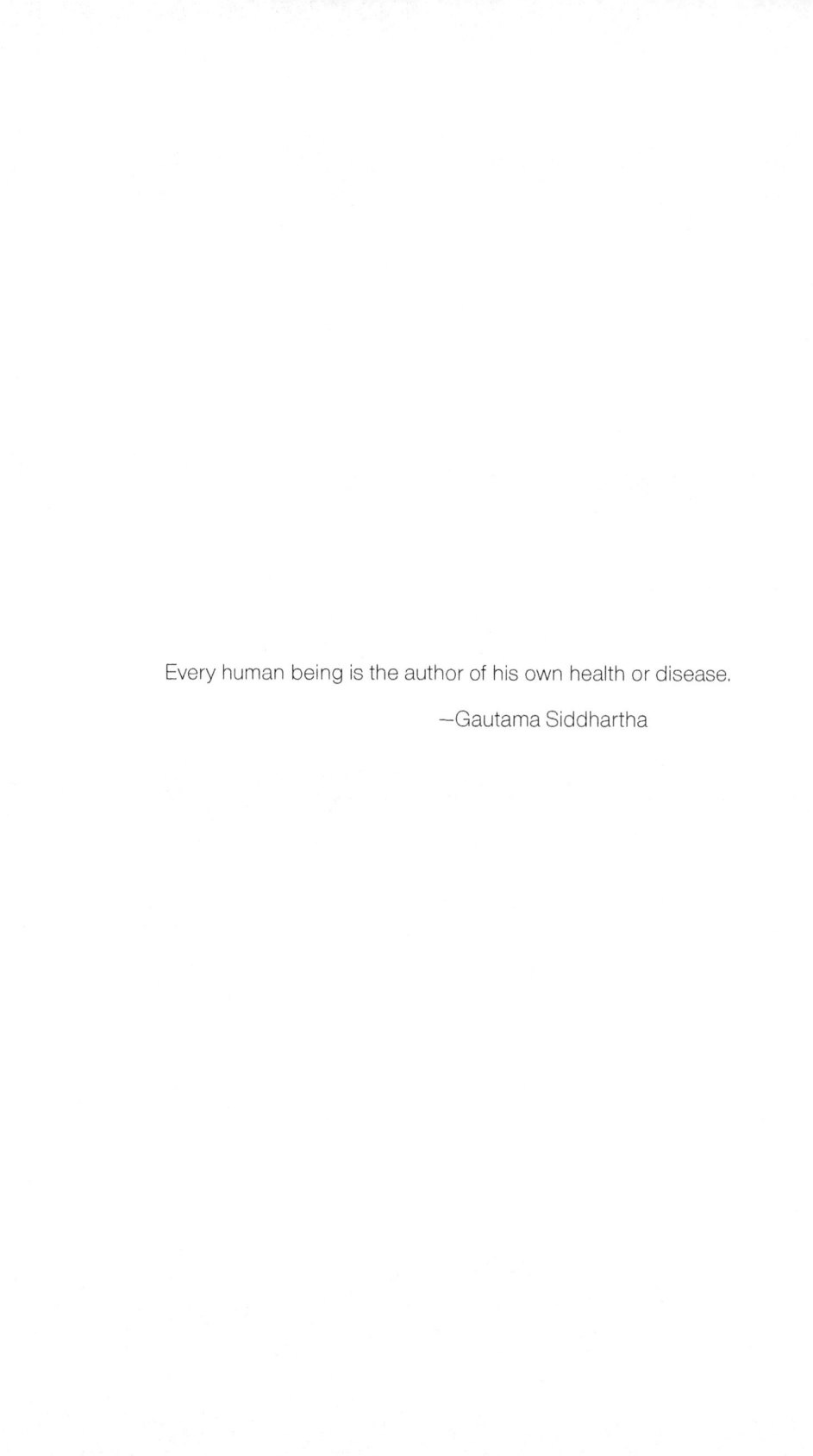

Every human being is the author of his own health or disease.

—Gautama Siddhartha

Dancing with Your Core Wound

> The journey between what you were and who you are now becoming; is where the Dance of Life really takes place.
>
> —Barbara DeAngelis

If you have followed me so far, something inside of you is now becoming inspired and interested in the exploration of the next step regarding your physical and personal healing. Could there be more to this already fascinating journey within? "Can I finally enter into unknown worlds I thought I would never see in my lifetime, like a deep-sea diver reaching far into the depth of unknown oceanic waters?"

Imagine you are the very first to discover this uncharted territory, as nobody so far has ever entered into such depths of our planet. This new world might evoke feelings of awe, wonder, amazement, a sense of being humble, or a sensation of belonging to a vast and boundless world offering limitless potentialities. You certainly will be deeply affected and changed by this experience. You might even feel inspired to change your current external life as you suddenly see and understand the very core of your Self, mirrored in the image of this journey. You might even get in touch with your commitment of your life's purpose and assignment as a result of your willingness to experience your conditioned behavioral expression of your mind and body. As you change, so will your dance!

Core Mind

We now know well that stress does not necessarily come from our external reality, but from the relationship and manner in which we experience it. Each behavior and expression of the experienced stress is completely unique and individual to our existence. It is our signature, like the distinct color or smell of a specific flower. It can't be duplicated as it belongs solely to us. Once we reach that level of our individual core, or center, of our mind and body, we will also see each and every aspect in our life illuminated and infiltrated by this unique theme or frequency. Our marriage, relationships, work environment, attitude to finances, connection to health and physical symptoms, and even the connection to our spiritual realm, will all be infused by this underlying constant inner behavioral pattern.

For many years during my professional career, I practiced more or less the conventional approach of classical homeopathy with the additional therapeutic tools of iridology and sclerology. Yet, over time, as I became distinctly aware of the deeper levels within my patients' psyches that were directly affecting their physical ailments, I found that within my consciousness and as a holistic physician I was no longer satisfied with the generally offered treatment protocols.

I have been blessed to know and work with many amazing teachers during my career. One of them, a pioneer of homeopathy, Dr. Rajan Sankaran, M.D. (Hom), expanded not only my own understanding of homeopathy, but was instrumental to my own healing path with his technique called the "Sensation Method." Sensation is the underlying individual pattern felt simultaneously in the mind and the body that eventually finds its way via our physical symptoms or disease. He also calls this pattern "The Other Song," which plays in parallel with our natural human song, our consciousness, and influences all aspects within our lives and circumstances. This inherent part of us is not to be confused with our subconscious mind, nor with our shadow, which I described earlier as storing our conditioned behaviors and belief systems, but explored through a completely different plane of experience altogether to reach far beyond both the subconscious and the conscious mind.

As mentioned earlier, we all describe our symptoms in a psychosomatic language. We speak of a "pounding" pain or of a "suffocating" relationship to an "unbearable" situation. Without being consciously aware, we choose words and sentences to describe our ailments that eventually lead us to this hidden realm, the core wound. Once we allow ourselves to touch and feel our deepest inner level, we not only use our descriptive language, but also gesticulate with hand movements the energetic image and frequency that rises like a lotus flower out of the mud from the very depth of our identity. At this point, we have gone far beyond our childhood stories, the blaming of our parents, or the lack of materialism. By becoming aware of our core and its unique expression, we can ultimately reduce its power and effect on our body. At this stage, we are becoming aware of the hidden aspects within ourselves. The actual experience of feeling this core frequency can then offer us the full potentiality of healing. At that point we are speaking about a radical transformation alongside the amelioration of physical symptoms.

This core experience doesn't adhere to the idea of space and time, or to our personal stories. It is an experience we remember, over and over, from past situations, and which we carry and express into our future events. This experience cannot be named; it cannot be labeled nor put into form, as it expresses itself from the deepest core of us through our individual realities.

As we live through intensely stressful situations, we often try to change our external environments in order to free ourselves from the seemingly external causes of stress. We may decide to leave the marriage or relationship, change jobs, or relocate to a new home. Perhaps, when we can't deal with the situation at all, we fall into depression or detach ourselves completely. If there is no immediate resolution, an individual might lean toward excessive consumption of alcohol or substance abuse, using them as an escape mechanism to avoid the stress. At this point, many of us will also choose self-help programs, read books, or join groups in the hopes that they will lead us back on the right track again. I joined an ashram in India.... Whatever works!

We constantly try to blame and project all our misery onto our external lives, making it, her, or him responsible for our circumstances. We see this dilemma particularly within marriages or intimate relationships. Here, the mirroring of our shadow is most heightened and on daily display, sometimes fueling the fire of projections to the point where life becomes a never-ending tennis match.

R. L., a 60-year-old woman, came to see me with vertigo attacks accompanied with nausea and vomiting. She'd had all the tests, but was told there was "no known cause." Allopathic medicine first suggested an inner ear problem, which was affecting her balance, but her ears were perfectly normal. She was prescribed the antibiotic Amoxicillin "just in case" there was an infection, but without improvement. R. L. describes her attacks as the feeling of "icy-coldness" throughout her body followed by the feeling of intense internal heat. These episodes are terrifying to her. She tells me that on the day of her first vertigo attack, she lived through a very dramatic disappointment, where she and two of her closest friends had a heated argument that resulted in the final dissolution of their friendship. In her words: "I felt so shaken up, overwhelmed, and in total shock to be treated like that. My whole world was shattered. I really blew to pieces, but knew I had to come to terms with it. I just wanted to curl up in my girlfriend's bed. That afternoon, I had my first attack and ended up in the hospital."

During the consultation, we explored R. L.'s experience and her feelings of mental and physical icy-coldness followed by the intense inner heat. The patient demonstrated to me with hand gestures what it felt like to experience this coldness within her body. As her hands trembled, I asked her to fall deeper into this experience by allowing mental images or other physical sensations to occur. Finally, she arrived at her childhood memories, which she freely shared. "My biggest wound is me feeling insecure. My father left when I was four years old, and I never felt safe with my mother. I even married my husband because he looked like my dad. I needed security and to feel safe. When he left, I was terrified! If anything happened to my mother, who would take care of me? Who would protect me? I need somebody around me; otherwise I feel disconnected."

When I asked her to further describe her sensation of feeling alone with no one to take care of her, she said, "There is a girl, she is in a dark room with no windows and no one knows she is there! As a young girl, I cried so much, over and over, but no one came to help me."

Core Mind

By the time she separated from her now ex-husband, R. L. was already experiencing minor panic attacks, feeling totally overwhelmed, waking up in the middle of the night feeling icy-cold with her teeth chattering, and experiencing a lot of fear. She was a single mother and was bringing up three children by herself.

The day of her first vertigo attack coincided with the falling-out with her two male friends, which had affected her deeply. The two represented safety and protection and were substitutes for her missing father. The vertigo attack was clearly a manifestation of a repeated pattern related to the initial shock experience of the loss of her father. Throughout her life, when a loved one separated from her, R. L. had physically reacted with internal icy coldness followed by intense heat, nausea, and vomiting. When she talked about her latest vertigo attack, she even expressed it as, "I lost my balance!"

As her friends represented a projected image of fatherhood for R. L., their "abandonment" left her feeling the same way she'd felt when her father had left her. Remember, the subconscious realm doesn't know time, and the tragic event of her friends' rejection caused the same deep emotional reaction her father's leaving had caused, as if he were leaving her for the very first time in her life. R. L.'s cellular body remembered that event when she'd been a child of four, when she'd displayed exactly the same symptoms of inner coldness followed by intense heat, chattering teeth, nausea, vomiting, and terror.

Beneath R. L.'s physical sensations lies a deep core wound, portrayed by the image of her being in a dark room without any windows where nobody comes to help her. This is an experience wrapped in a haze of total terror in which she felt abandoned and forsaken. These feelings represent R. L.'s core wound and are the very sensations mirrored in every aspect of her life and running through these aspects like a continuous red thread.

R. L.'s vertigo would only pass or be ameliorated if treated with appropriate natural remedies like homeopathy and natural supplementation and through awareness and acknowledgment of her core belief of deep abandonment.

Core Mind

I have so far presented two cases with vertigo symptomatology, yet you can clearly see that each case focuses on a completely different story relative to initial events and thus demand individually tailored treatments. To prescribe a generalized prescription for vertigo would not result in lasting amelioration.

This process is not an intellectual or analytical exercise, but an act of deeply allowing oneself to feel the depth of one's belief system. In homeopathy, we call this core belief system a *delusion*. Although admittedly temporarily stressful, R. L.'s chronic underlying stress is not due to the vertigo with its symptomatic picture, but is and always will be the delusion and fear of being abandoned at any time, at any moment. It is the theme that runs her show, so to speak. As soon as R. L. recognizes her physical sensations of icy-cold and intense heat are important pointers to, or links from, her delusion, the symptoms, including the vertigo, should begin to recede. At that point, she will stop feeling like a victim of the situation and consciously become an active participant in her own healing process. Remember, whatever your experience, it is not limited to your specific situation, but applies to you as a whole and for most of your life. This experience is who you are, and it will remain the source of your constant stress until you address it.

As we continue to evolve in our consciousness and look at the possibilities for healing ourselves and the planet, we are ultimately asked to transcend this level to recognize our delusions, to enter and touch the space in between, the space of energy and all-encompassing source. When we do, we are able to transmute both polarities of our self-inflicted belief systems and our learned defense mechanisms. Then, we are truly free!

Again, in R. L.'s case, her delusion was represented by her two friends' desertion, but it was not they or the situation that had created her stress. It had been created by the way she perceived and reacted to this reality. This was her dis-ease, which was totally unique and individual to her. Her stress was inseparable from her individuality. Here again, psychotherapy or counseling would be beneficial to help her understand the connection of her vertigo to the loss of her father at an early age. Such an analysis would still be based on an analytical and intellectual explanation, however, rather than the actual effect of the experience of having lost her father. When my patient realizes the inherent pattern of her reactions to the totality of all her stress situations, she will eventually be able to live a life with less stress, a life free of its self-repeating drama. My patient's truth is reflected in the depth and totality of her entire experience.

The trained homeopath is not interested in the question of why something happened, but in the deeper understanding of what happened to the patient while he or she was experiencing that external circumstance. The practitioner is interested in the individual expression of the patient's behavior. In this way, because each expression of delusion is unique and individual, any possibility for projection regarding case taking or case analysis is essentially annihilated, for both the patient and the practitioner.

Rajan Sankaran in *The Other Song* writes: "We need to realize that part of the essence of the concepts in this work lies in the notion that our behavior and our feelings stem from something much deeper in our beings. They are rooted in a very basic, inexplicable experience unique to each one of us. This experience is not emotional or intellectual; it is a sensation felt in the body and minds simultaneously, one that is constant, and one that colors our whole experience of life. This sensation is our constant companion, the 'Other Song' that keeps singing within us."

Illness mirrors an expression of a learned behavior given birth during a very stressful situation in the past. Imagine that someone had a car accident and a red van was involved. Now, years later, whenever he sees a red van on the road passing by he feels an actual physical, cellular memory within his body that reminds him of his past accident and causes him to sweat and have heart palpitations and for his emotional body to activate with anxiety. Do you see how this can happen? To truly heal these dormant cellular behaviors takes time, patience, and a willingness to gently open the lid of one's inner Pandora's box. It is a process and a journey, but one that certainly can become the most enriching and transformative dance of one's life.

Core Mind

I'd like to explain now in more detail the concept of Sensation Method relative to my personal story. In this way, you may be able to apply these principles to your own personal situation more easily.

My last severe episode of intense physical pain started in the year 2004. At that time, I was teaching at the local university, taking care of my patients, working as director of a children's foundation, struggling in the midst of a long and drawn out legal situation involving multiple attorneys, and often feeling upset about not being able to spend enough time with my children (as I was living in another country). You could say that I was extremely stressed! I had over time become aware of a left-sided abdominal pain that was now giving me stabbing and burning sensations. As I was busy and a workaholic by nature (pushing through life), I had ignored the initial signs, thinking that by taking a few natural supplements it would all go away. Even a skilled and natural physician can sometimes be ignorant about her own body! Initially this approach actually succeeded in ameliorating the pain. It also helped that during this time I entered into a new relationship. I was in love and happy.

After six months into the relationship, however, the abdominal pains came back. This time, the pains were much stronger than ever before. I was also realizing that the relationship wasn't as "easy" as I'd initially imagined it would be, and that the stressful circumstances in which I found myself were affecting me more and more deeply. I tried to heal my physical pains with all the tools in my remedy toolbox. This time, though, there was no lasting and beneficial result. By now, my entire lower abdomen was filled with multiple kinds of pains. Some were cutting, like a knife, some singed like fire, and some just left me achy and sore. Quite often I felt myself on the verge of literally passing out from the on-going intensity. I flew thousands of miles to find any medical diagnosis I could, from the U.S. to the UK and back again, spending thousands of dollars on medical bills. From the gastroenterologist, gynecologist, to oncologist, I tried every possible route to get to the bottom of my ailments. I consulted Native American shamanic healers to several faith healers with their strange and often unusual techniques. In the meantime, my pains were reaching an unbearable crescendo day and night.

Core Mind

The allopathic medical side established the diagnosis of diverticulitis, blocked fallopian tubes, ovarian cysts, congested uterus, and endometriosis ... all the way to possible neoplasm, meaning cancer. Several ultrasounds indicated a large mass that often, strangely, disappeared in between procedures. Another diagnosis was irritable bowel syndrome (IBS) caused by a stressful life. The last diagnosis was that it was "all in my mind," as no absolutely clear cause could really be found.

According to the iridology and sclerology findings in my eyes, I knew that I had diverticulitis with toxic biofilms, which had attached themselves to my colon. At that time, to meet such a challenge was totally over my head and professional capacity, as I was so wrapped up in this living nightmare that I'd lost all objectivity. As the months went by, I developed peritonitis. Suppurating pus was now leaking through and out of my body and detrimentally affecting my ovaries and uterus. I knew then that I was seriously heading downhill with my ailing body and in need of instant help.

The process of numerous hospital visits began, followed by three abdominal surgeries. The first two included the partial removal of my female organs; the third and final one was a total hysterectomy. By then, it was hard to envision that I would survive a third surgery. Emotionally, I felt so disappointed as I watched my body being butchered, cut, and violently invaded. And being a doctor of natural medicine didn't help at all; in fact, it exacerbated the situation even more, as all my acquired medical knowledge literally went out the window.

How did I feel throughout this time? Feelings of anger, rage, resentment, grief, disappointment, and being a victim of it all roamed inside of me constantly. Aside from the ongoing pain, I also was faced with coming to terms with having lost my ability to bear children while at the same time being thrown instantly into a raging menopause.

As I intend that my story should serve you as a learning example and as a guide in understanding the core of my sensations and delusions, at this point if you had asked me, "How does it feel, experiencing all these feelings and dealing with all these different treatments at the same time?" my immediate answer would have been, "These pains are controlling me. I can't be free anymore. I can't be myself anymore. I am literally barely surviving each and every day. I have lost all joy in my life. I can't push through this anymore, and I can't change the situation. I want to be free again, *me* again!"

It is easy to see that my chosen words and language in describing my belief system regarding my illness were focused on feeling controlled, feeling denied the right to be me (the pains) and of being robbed of my joy to live, as well as feeling a total lack of control in resolving the situation. Remember, my initial story started with my controlled childhood and upbringing, and my living for years in solitude and isolation.

My current life was filled with many stressful situations, including too much work, accumulating relationship problems, and the emotional suppression of missing my children. Needless to say, I felt as if I were on the verge of an upcoming explosion. My body was trying to tell me, over and over again, that my mind, my emotions, and my relationship had reached a serious momentum of crisis, yet I couldn't see or understand its message. My body and I were in serious conflict here, and by relating to *The Pain* as something outside of me, or something that was controlling me; I was becoming more and more separate from my body. It had become a vicious cycle.

As I felt utterly controlled and overwhelmed, my defense mechanism was to control every aspect of my life even more conscientiously. I criticized my partner, followed countless treatment protocols, read all the appropriate books, spent hours on the Internet, evaluated my own blood tests, and continuously changed my diet regime. As nothing seemed to work, these tasks only contributed to turning me into a desperate and angry woman. I criticized and scolded doctors, as well as holistic physicians, about their incompetence and inability to heal me.

The pain was now so bad that I was unable to control it anymore and unable to "push through it" to go beyond this phase of my life. Of course, it was then that my emotional state counteracted with my already presenting abdominal symptoms by exacerbating their intensity.

I took a rainbow of painkillers from mild to heavy potencies without any relief. An arsenal of homeopathic remedies earned me only brief hours of sleep, and my belly began to show the brown burn marks from applying hot water bottles months at a time. I was desperate!

As I went through my library searching for answers, I revisited the book *Anatomy of Spirit* by Caroline Myss, Ph.D., which speaks about the chakra system, the body's seven centers of spiritual and physical power based on the Hindu tradition. In reading her material, I began to understand that my second chakra (located in my lower abdomen), the place of all my physical symptoms, was related to the subject of the power of relationships. This energy wheel comes alive around the age of seven. At this age, children start to interact with other children and adults to learn about the concept of relationship in general. Due to my unusual childhood of living in isolation, this natural process of learning how to cultivate relationships was significantly underdeveloped. During this time, my father had left the family unit as well.

The second chakra resonates to the general need for relationships with other people and in counterpoint with the need to control one's physical environment. The illness that is birthed in this center is activated by the fear of losing control. Caroline Myss points out that the second chakra's primary fear is the fear of losing control *or* being controlled by another through the dominating power of events or conditions such as addiction, rape, betrayal, impotence, financial loss, and abandonment by our primary partner or professional colleagues. It also represents the fear of the loss of power of the physical body.

All of these examples were part of my emotional scenario and physical crisis. At this point, there was no doubt that the totality of my illness was based on my belief system of being controlled and dominated, either by people, circumstances, or physical pain, and not only by the imminently occurring events. As there are always two sides to a coin, there also existed a second viewpoint regarding my depleted second chakra. The primary strength of this energy center is based on the ability and stamina to survive financially and physically on one's own, as well as to defend and protect oneself. The meaning of the second chakra is represented by the sentiment "honor one another," no matter the circumstances. Therefore, the presented lessons and my personal evolution were dependent on my honoring myself as a person, woman, and mother. It was also about my learning how to protect myself by saying no and by honoring the people in my surrounding environment.

Caroline Myss explains the second chakra like this: "The challenge of the second chakra is to learn what motivates us to make the choices we do. In learning about our motivations, we learn about the content of our spirits. Are you filled with fear, or are you filled with faith? Every choice we make contains the energy of either faith or fear, and the outcome of every decision reflects to some extent that faith or fear."

My complete and transformative healing required the vital ingredient of making responsible choices regarding all my decisions and actions in life, acts which would allow me to transcend the conditioned and perceived dualistic concept of division between others and myself. As long as I was acting from fear of being controlled or trying to control my environment or another person, I was only keeping my inner conflict alive. It was time to end this drama.

Needless to say, my relationship ended, I reduced my workload, and decided to thoroughly dedicate my life to my healing journey. I acknowledged that I had never really touched the core of my limited belief pattern before, despite all the years of therapies and holistic treatments. I also knew that one day I would have to go there!

We now fully understand that not the name of the disease, its label, its description, or even its recognized belief system will ultimately shift or heal the physical pathology. Here, we have to go a step deeper into the realm of our sensations. Again, in my case, the next questions would then be: Can you describe the sensation, the experience of being controlled? What does it feel like?

When you ask someone to answer a question based on the description of the sensations that underlie his belief system, you often observe a moment of silence, a moment where you can witness the struggle between mind and body. To experience the sensations that have created one's belief system is a *process*, one that goes beyond the mind, as it has ceased to grasp or control the aftermath of that experience. In this moment, if we let ourselves, we drop or fall into a world of the senses and are able to describe our story from the place of the depths of our subconscious mind.

Core Mind

For me, the feeling of "being controlled" was experienced as an extremely tight physical sensation accompanied by cramps and pressing pain. Although I often felt paralyzed by these sensations, I also, contrarily, felt the need to employ my willpower relentlessly to push through (for me, the opposite reaction to feeling tight) the current or past challenging circumstances in my life. When describing my emotional tightness, I simultaneously felt my tight and cramping intestines. As I entered the realm where I felt the tightness, which was like a spastic hand contorted by rigid and ongoing constriction, I instantly realized the connection between my core wound and my physical symptoms. It was in that moment that my whole life fell into place and years of agony began to make sense! I realized that I had experienced countless stressful situations in the past as external forms of oppression and control, as a kind of energy field that was continuously "pushing" against my will. These oppressive forces took the form of my partner and the conflict that arose from being a mother and having a career. It was also lodged in my health, the relationship to my nutritional intake, and my physical pain.

For the first time, I became the witness to my reactions regarding my control issues, which not only had always been automatic, instant, without rational thought, but mostly out of proportion to the actual presenting reality. Once I understood this fact, I was guided to the most appropriate homeopathic remedy based on the core principle of domination and control. As I allowed myself to deeply see and feel my automatic response of my belief system and the possibilities available to me by fundamentally changing its behavior, my body slowly started to heal, relax, and find its joy again.

My own story and those of my patients clearly illustrate that we are not only affected by our external circumstances, but by our individual perception of these events. The external reality is not typically the cause of our stress; rather it is our perception of reality that is ultimately the deciding factor in our health or disease. This is the very reason why our cellular biology changes its behavioral pattern according to its influencing environment, whether the external one or the inner psychological one; it is not due to our genealogy. It is the perception of the carrier that determines the behavior of his cells.

Core Mind

Our delusions are not born in our mind, nor do they arise from our emotions. They are born from a place deep within us, beyond our intellect and rationality. To sense and feel our belief systems we have to enter a world deep within, a world of many discoveries and wonders. Our stress in life is not a cause-and-effect phenomenon, but a mirror, an external trigger that stimulates our inherent behavioral structures. In Oprah Winfrey's words: "Turn your wounds into wisdom." Every experience in life is not created by the situation itself, but by your perception and relationship toward it.

Once I really admitted to myself that I was seeing everything and everybody in my life through colored glasses that convinced me I was being controlled, oppressed, or rejected, I also began to compassionately understand my physical reactions to these situations as well. Each event was related, regardless of form or shape, with the same result, where I felt one of two reactions: I either felt controlled or free. There was no in-between.

The Sensation Method of Dr. Rajan Sankaran offers many more layers and findings on this subject. While his book doesn't serve as a homeopathic textbook, it can serve as a tool and healing method regarding the understanding of our mind. If you would like to learn more about these tools, please refer to them individually.

As I explored my wholeness with self-acceptance and self-love for the "ALL I AM," a newfound peace entered my life to penetrate each fiber of my mind, body, and soul like an unmistakably sweet fragrance. The imperative truth that peace cannot be attained in the outer world without touching and living our inner peace became more and more apparent to me. Although simple to understand intellectually, it is a complicated concept to integrate, and one often beyond our current ability to sustain.

As I am finishing this chapter, Canadian Oscar-winning director James Cameron has just resurfaced after diving to the Challenger Deep, the deepest known point in the Earth's sea floor hydrosphere in the Mariana Trench of the western section of the Pacific Ocean. During his solo dive, Cameron was completely isolated from the rest of the world, and commented: "I feel like I literally, in the space of one day, have gone to another planet and come back."

Core Mind

This is the experience you will touch inside yourself once you have deeply felt your core mind and its related physical sensations. It is like stepping into another world, yet being fully conscious of your presence and your body. As there are no coincidences in life, the story of James Cameron's first deep-sea dive reflects the synchronicity of our willingness and maturity toward our own inner deep-sea journeys to wellness. As he touched upon a world never before visited, so will you touch upon an inner world never before seen by your inner or outer eyes.

༄

The night has drawn to its close, the dance rests in stillness, and you and your partner have arrived at a place of peace and non-movement. Right now, you both decide to take a break. As you leave the dance floor under the black night sky, your hearts are filled with a deep sense of gratitude. You both acknowledge this moment of profound transformation in each of you and as a couple. This dance poured through all your veins, like rushing water from a waterfall, drenching your essence with a completely new perception to whatever will happen from now on.

A primal instinct, an inner voice, speaking through both of you, announces the next phase of your journey to freedom. This time, you will separate from each other and learn to dance by yourself. The next phase will become your own dance, free of any external dependency or tangible source. It is time to learn to dance by yourself, so you can fully feel and get to know your body. It is time to step onto your dance floor alone.

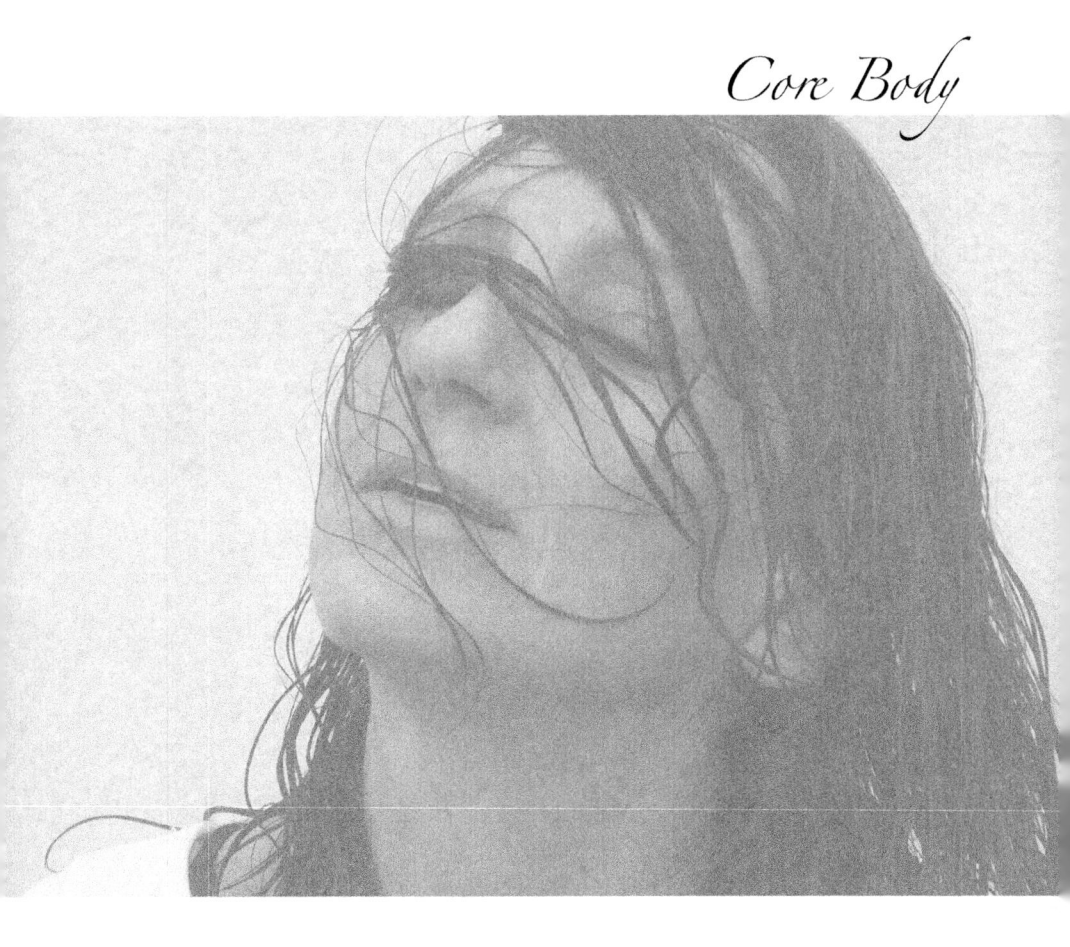

Core Body

When you step further into the story you came to live, not only does the mythic territory open, but the deep self moves and the world of imagination and meaning comes toward you.

—Michael Meade

Toxicity Dances through the Body

> To dance is to pray
> To pray is to heal
> To heal is to give
> To give is to live
> To live is to dance.
>
> —MariJo Moore

It is late afternoon and you walk alone along the sandy beach of a tropical island. The air is still filled with the day's glowing warmth and your skin and body is soaking in the last sunrays of this magical place. As the grainy sand kisses your feet, you softly glance over the endless horizon. The beach invites itself as your treasure chest, with beautiful shells, curly seaweed, washed-up driftwood and the scattered fallen branches of palm trees. A slight breeze tousles your hair, which you gently brush to the side, as you taste the salty skin on your cheek. Life is calm, you are calm, and this day feels just perfect.

As you walk along the quiet coastline, your ears catch some sounds that seem to come from the far distance. As you walk closer to their place of origin, you recognize a gathering of some locals drumming with joy to the soon setting sun. For some reason you feel mesmerized by the intensity of the dark-brown and sun-kissed dancing hands moving up and down on their drums and filling the air with the palpable rhythm of your heart. The beats are strong and slowly enter your body, allowing you to sway to their rhythm. Your fingers start tapping on your thighs and your toes wriggle themselves into the soft sand. Your body wants and has to move now ... and it does! As you fall into the arms of the beating sound, you forget the beach, the people, the sand, and even the ocean you just admired a moment ago. You and the body are merging with the rhythm of the drums. There is nothing to do, there are no thoughts, there is no you as you merge and disappear into this moment of sound. Are you ready to feel and fully explore your body?

In the previous chapter, you became aware of the deep interconnectedness of your thoughts, emotions, and belief systems filtering through your cells with their respective associated behavior to your life experience. Holistic medicine always emphasizes the concept of the totality of the body as it interacts with its organs, tissue, nerves, bones, and fluids. Any effect on one part of the body affects the other parts as well, as each part in your body has an important impact on the whole body. Your body is the most magnificent instrument on Earth! With millions of functions and chemical processes occurring each and every day, it supersedes any technological invention today. Your body is the most exquisite and efficiently engineered masterpiece, and is vitalized and fueled by your highest intelligence.

Did you know that it takes 200 muscles to take one step; that a pair of human feet contains 250,000 sweat glands; that the acid in your stomach is strong enough to dissolve razor blades; or that the human brain cell can hold five times as much information as the Encyclopedia Britannica? Did you also know that the average red blood cell lives for only 120 days? There are 2.5 trillion (give or take) red blood cells in your body at any moment. To maintain this number, about 2.5 million new ones need to be produced every second by your bone marrow. That's like a new population of the city of Toronto every second. A red blood cell can circumnavigate your body in less than 20 seconds. Your body has about 5.6 liters (6 quarts) of blood. These 5.6 liters of blood circulate

Core Body

through the body three times every minute. In 24 hours, the blood in the body travels a total of 12,000 miles— that's four times the width of North America.

Considering all the tissues and cells in the body, 25 million new cells are being produced each second. That's a little less than the population of Canada—every second! Nerve impulses travel at over 400 kilometers (25 miles per hour). Our heart beats around 100,000 times every day. Our eyes can distinguish up to 1 million color surfaces and take in more information than the largest telescope known to man. Our lungs inhale over 2 million liters of air every day and are large enough to cover a tennis court. In 1 square inch of your hand, you will find 9 feet of blood vessels, 600 pain sensors, 9,000 nerve endings, 36 heat sensors, and 75 pressure sensors. And this is just the beginning!

In order to function at its optimal health, your body needs to be able to communicate with you, just as your cells need to communicate with each other. This sharing of information is vitally important for the overall well-being of your body. Today, this phenomenon of "talking to each other" has been severely disrupted, not only by our attitude and relationship to our bodies, but by an overwhelming accumulated cellular toxicity affecting our cell membranes, which are then unable to receive or provide nutrients to their overall host. Your body is a superb example of well-organized teamwork. Your choice regarding the quality of your life and environment to which you expose your body determines its inner functions and well-being. Each externally and internally perceived stimulus profoundly influences this ingenious system of cellular teamwork.

※

Let's embark on a scenic sightseeing tour within the body, travelling from organ to organ by getting to know its functions and miracle tasks. In my role as a teacher, I always incorporate the fascinating information regarding the theme called the TOXIC STRESS CYCLE, which is fundamentally a process of "passing the buck" of accumulated toxins; in other words, a pathway through the body through compensation whereby stress is passed on from one body system to another. This domino effect, starting at your daily plate of food, travels throughout your body only to complete its full circle at your digestive system again. The Toxic Stress Cycle shapes itself as a perpetual stress pattern and can only be broken with natural and well-chosen nutrients, as well as a conscious and life-affirming mindset.

Dr. Ben Collimore, who also was a student of Dr. Wheelwright, initially formulated the term "Toxic Stress Cycle." I was fortunate to learn about this invaluable information from Dr. Jack Tips. All the following chapters about the Core Body are gratefully dedicated to his brilliance and his mastership of integrative medicine.

Your Dance Starts and Ends with Your Digestive System

All illness starts with your digestion—or lack of it. Your digestive system is the very first entrance door of your present and future diseases in your life. Our food is our medicine and our medicine is our food. A simple statement, so often overlooked, yet with profound repercussions on our health. Because what we choose to eat today will show up tomorrow as the picture of our health. Poor digestion or an imbalanced diet is the start and end of the self-feeding Toxic Stress Cycle. Simply put, what you eat determines your life and your death.

When was the last time you sat down at the table feeling a sense of wonder by looking at the intense green of a lightly steamed broccoli or smelling the intoxicating aroma of a fresh ginger root? When was the last time you remember taking the time to chew and taste your food? When was the last time you remember enjoying a Sunday morning breakfast with your friends? When was the last time you remember stuffing yourself with a sandwich while rushing to get the next train home from work? Our fast and over-stimulated lives, primarily focused on speed, time, and production, do not allow us to live in synchronicity with the body or the digestive system. Did you know that your digestive system is really a nervous system, encased by the general nervous

Core Body

system and autonomic nervous system? Whatever you feel affects your stomach, intestines, and/or colon.

Your DIGESTIVE SYSTEM is made up of the digestive tract, a series of hollow organs joined in a long, twisting tube from the mouth to the anus, and other organs, like the pancreas, liver, gallbladder, and kidneys that help the body break down and absorb food. It also includes endocrine glands like the hypothalamus, the master gland situated in the brain that directs and influences your digestion.

Imbalances of this system are mainly created by a general lack of enzymes, improper mastication (chewing), the lack of nerve flow from the spine, organs pushing or impinging on each other, or improper food combinations from either too much food or poor food choices. An irregular eating schedule, for example, where one eats late at night, can also produce imbalance. Not to mention the exposure to chemical food additives, excessive use of microwaves, fried foods, and drinking excessive beverages with meals. All these factors, and many more, can cause the production of toxins, which are then passed on to the overall system, including the blood stream, to result in major stress to the tissues within the body. To be part of a healthy and efficient digestive system requires the best nutrition comprised of a balanced ratio of proteins, carbohydrates, and oils in the form of organic and fresh produce. I will talk about a good life-sustaining diet more in the next chapters.

Interestingly, the digestive system can be compared to the way the brain works. The brain takes in external stimulants and digests them so we can receive its filtered information via our consciousness. The digestive system takes in external stimulants, like food, and breaks it down into suitable particles, which can then be assimilated back into our system. Here, the digestion focuses on tangible substances, the discrimination of beneficial or toxic elements, the assimilation of beneficial materials, as well as the excretion, or elimination, of waste products. However, both processes are really quite similar.

Digestive imbalances are often caused by emotional disturbances, as revealed by our chosen language and verbal expressions in describing them. We state our likes and dislikes as "This is not to my taste" or our aggressive behavior as "I am getting my teeth into it" or facing unbearable situations as "I find this hard to swallow." A grieving person experiences a lump in the throat; a depressed person might say, "This is hard to digest." An introvert might swallow his anger or someone very upset might say, "I am getting eaten up inside." The basic tendency to withhold our feelings and aggressions and turn them inward and against us can lead to the degeneration of stomach tissue or an ulcer. Rather than expressing our emotions freely, we are often digesting ourselves!

Ask yourself: *What is eating me up? What issue is so difficult to swallow? What am I so sour about?* If we leave the stomach area and go further along the intestines, we might find the individual suffering from diarrhea. Then the practitioner might be interested to know more about the mental and emotional components regarding this presenting symptom. In this case, the patient might voice: "I am scared shitless!" Can you see the relationship from the mind to the body?

And how about somebody who suffers from chronic constipation who says, "I can't let go off this dreadful relationship!" Or the diabetic with an inability to produce insulin or assimilate sugar who has difficulty enjoying the sweetness of life and is therefore in need of compensating with some substitute "sweetness."

Once the STOMACH is unable to clear the ingested toxins, it will pass them on to the small and large intestines, THE COLON. Here, the incomplete digestion, as well as the toxic overload, results in the fermentation and putrefaction of food particles—that is, your food starts to rot in your body. When our bowel flora colonizes with the most beneficial bacterial cultures these situations are usually resolved, yet in today's world even these natural processes have become severely out of balance. Our colon's flora should be around 85% beneficial bacteria, such as lactobacillus, bifidus, bulgaricus and other strains, and around 15% potentially harmful bacteria, such as coliform, streptococcus, and so forth. However, due to our unhealthy diet and overuse of antibiotics, most often this ratio is now reversed, leaving us with 85% harmful bacteria and only 15% beneficial bacteria. Our imbalanced intestinal bowel flora influences diseases like dysbiosis, a condition of microbial imbalance, which can lead to the now common "leaky gut syndrome" and other man-made diseases of today's over-stimulated lifestyle. When our intestines are affected, we are unable to absorb vital nutrients, leaving us depleted of converted energy, which we desperately need in order to stay alive.

New research studies have shown that as newborns find their way through the mother's birth canal during the birthing process, they gather beneficial bacteria via the placenta and the vagina's skin that colonize the mother's digestive system in the womb. Although identified as "bacteria," these microbes are uniquely designed for the well-being of the newborn's life, serving, for example, as precursors for the baby's healthy and fully functional digestive system.

All plants, animals, and humans live in close association with microbial organisms. Up until relatively recently, however, the interactions of plants and animals with the microbial world have been defined mostly in the context of disease states. Only a relatively small number of studies have acknowledged its beneficial symbiosis with our bodies, particularly the digestive system. But organisms do not live in isolation. Microbes have evolved in the context of complex communities. Their presence and functions are incredibly important to our optimal health, but can only thrive if we offer them a well-balanced inner terrain—in this case, a balanced bowel flora.

Our cells and we are not designed to live in isolation; we never have been. Today, we are aware that the totality of microbes, called microbiome, which represent genetic elements interacting within a particular environment, from our digestive system to the soil, seawater and freshwater, are vital parts of a symbiotic and self-sustaining totality, within our bodies or the planet as a whole. Here, one ecosystem serves and feeds the other. Bacterial mutual relationships are crucial for our survival, and an imbalanced gut flora can lead to a number of different disorders.

Although bacteria are often associated with infections, these uniquely designed bacteria that colonize the body's surface, the skin, and the inside of our bodies are essential for life. We are dependent on them to help digest our food, produce certain vitamins, regulate our immune system, and keep us healthy by protecting us against other disease-causing bacteria. Imbalances have been linked to various disorders from irritable bowel syndrome to obesity. Altered microbiomes may even have an effect on personality and autism.

As we learn more about the significance of our relationship and attitude to life and ourselves, both of which influence our cellular behavior, we can also see how the mother's lifestyle during her pregnancy is linked to the first bacterial communities that develop in a fetus. It is interesting to note that the first bacteria that colonize the newborn's gut are thought to influence the bacterial species that follow it. For example, if the mother consumes an organic diet during her pregnancy or is a heavy smoker, her behavior will determine the kind of acquired bacteria that will affect the newborn's susceptibility to future illnesses like asthma or eczema. What we eat and how we live not only influences our body, but the bodies of many future generations to come. At this point in time, we cannot afford to continue living in ignorance anymore, as the repercussions will only heavily ricochet on us.

I highly recommend introducing fermented food into your daily diet. Fermented foods serve as significant nutrients in balancing the diversity of bacteria of the digestive system. Only in the recent past have fermented foods begun to disappear from our plate. Modern pickles and sauerkraut are made with vinegar instead of the traditional method of lacto-fermentation, which uses salt. Bread and pasta are made with commercial yeast instead of natural leavening products like wild yeast (sourdough). Wine, beer, and cheeses are pasteurized, a process that kills off all the good bacteria we so desperately need to maintain optimal health. Fermenting food is nature's natural excellence and humans all over the world have been utilizing the technique since ancient times. (For further information, refer to books like *The Body Ecology Diet* by Donna Gates and Linda Schatz or *The Art of Fermentation* by Sandor Ellis Katz and Michael Pollan.)

Culinary author Sandor Katz describes fermented food in this way: "In the normal scheme of things, we'd never have to think twice about replenishing the bacteria that allow us to digest food. But since we're living with antibiotic drugs and chlorinated water and antibacterial soap and all these factors in our contemporary lives that I'd group together as a 'war on bacteria,' if we fail to replenish [good bacteria], we won't effectively get nutrients out of the food we're eating."

And so our bucket, filled with toxins, already handed from the stomach to the intestines, is now passed on to the LIVER and GALLBLADDER. If there can be said to be a most important organ in the body, in many ways the liver would be it. In some ways, it is even more important than the heart. As the body's main natural detoxifier, it has a huge effect not only on our mental and emotional states, but also on our physical health and longevity in its role of removing poisons and metabolic waste products. From food processing and agricultural chemicals, environmental pollutants, vaccinations, prescription and recreational drugs, dental fillings, radiation to junk food, we rely on the liver to take care of processing all of it. Next to cleansing our blood, the liver stores vitamins and minerals, takes care of hormones, is responsible for the metabolism of proteins, constructs 50,000 systems of enzymes to govern metabolic activity throughout the body, and neutralizes anything harmful—and these are only some of its functions. The liver stores and generates energy; it processes proteins and it detoxifies. Both foreign poisons and those produced by the body itself are deactivated and made soluble in the liver so that they can be excreted via the gallbladder or the kidneys. The liver is not only one of the largest organs in the human body, but its central organ. It is the body's finest laboratory!

When the toxins from your colon enter your portal system, your liver and gallbladder are affected. These toxins, gases, and chemicals are now traveling from the colon to your liver, only to contribute to the liver's already heavy workload. Now the liver becomes overworked, as it has to deal with its own thousands of functions along with the accumulated waste from your digestive system. We call this having a congested liver.

Did you know when your eyesight begins to weaken that your liver is directly related to the process? When the liver is overloaded, eyesight is immediately affected. In fact, patients often notice an improvement of their vision after a good liver cleanse. There is also a direct relationship between the left liver lobe and seasonal allergies attacks. Due to the excess accumulation of toxins and the liver's inability to detoxify incoming proteins, particularly in the left liver lobe, seasonal allergies return year after year despite all the over-the-counter prescribed medication you may take. If you want to heal your environmental allergies or food sensitivities, choose the liver as your prime candidate for where to start any treatment.

Despite the phenomenal amount of work the liver can do, there are limits to what it can accomplish. Organs and glands that have an impaired ability to rebuild are then prone to infection and depleted immune system . . . which leads us to a situation where the cells, in this case liver cells, begin to exhibit destructive behavior. The environment inside us, as outside of us, determines the behavioral response of our cells. This principle applies to your Mind, Body, and Soul throughout.

Did you know that your lifelong constipation might be linked to the strong possibility of a sluggish liver, not just a lazy colon? Constipation has little to do with the need for laxatives, but has everything to do with an overworked and congested liver. And it is not just your colon that is affected here, but also your entire bloodstream, carrying these "unwanted shopping bags" filled with waste.

The Healing Triad of STOMACH, COLON, and LIVER is the fundamental and essential block of interdependent and interrelated functions of optimal health. If these three aspects are well balanced and nourished, you will experience vitality, a smooth detoxification throughout all your body systems, and a joyful, rejuvenating well-being. It is therefore of vital importance that your regular maintenance of your body includes the daily attention to these three critical organs.

Symbolically, the liver manifests as the capacity to distinguish and clearly evaluate all aspects in your life. This process of clear thinking and being able to make the most appropriate decisions is fundamentally interrupted if the liver cannot detoxify the body's own produced metabolic waste products and incoming unprocessed toxins. I have often noticed after completing a liver cleanse the wonderful by-product of unusually clear and sharp thought processes, including the ability to arrive at clear decisions despite some emotional stagnation. During stressful times, we might say, "I can't make a decision right now; this is all too overwhelming for me!" This is your liver talking here, because it really wants you to know that it is not just the mind that is overworked, but also your physical body and its liver cells.

A sick liver shows us that we are taking in more of something than we can possibly cope with. It is a sign that our world has taken on an immoderate and exaggerated lifestyle of too much food and/or too much rich food, alcohol, and perhaps excess drugs, all of which influence our ability for clear judgment and for evaluating what's right or wrong. With a clean and fully functional liver, you will be surprised how much easier it will be to make effective and appropriate decisions again.

Another aspect of an imbalanced liver can be seen in people with exaggerated and inflated egos. These "liver types" may have an air of quiet self-possession, stability, and detachment that inspire respect, but typically carry a strong sense of inadequacy. They tend to be intellectual with a conservative outlook, and often hold prestigious positions as diplomats, executives, lawyers, and doctors. Many of these individuals are actually deeply insecure, however, exaggerating the truth to bolster their low self-esteem. They often resist change, since challenges cause great apprehension or anxiety. In general, they have a distinguished, almost haughty appearance to disguise their deep-seated lack of confidence, often unseen by the outside world. Needless to say, liver types display digestive disturbances with excess flatulence, expressing their inflated egos throughout their lower abdomens.

If you are suffering from liver problems, then it is time to ask yourself the following questions: Are there any areas in my life where I have lost my capacity to clearly assess and evaluate? Where is my keen sense of distinguishing between what is healthy and good for me and what is toxic in my life? Do I feel confident in life? Do I appear overconfident by trying to hide my lack of self-esteem?

The GALLBLADDER is intimately linked to the liver as it collects the yellow bile that is produced by the liver from cholesterol. The bile flows from the gallbladder into the digestive system, where it processes all the lipid (oil) particles of your diet. When the bile duct is obstructed, complications often arise in the form of gallstones.

My biological father never really got over his divorce and separation from my mother. More than 40 years later, he was still harboring a bitter resentment about their dissolved marriage. The gallbladder with its bitter bile is directly related to the emotion of withheld and acerbic resentment. My father expressed just such an embittered nature, which ultimately resulted in gallstones' blocking his duct. His symptomatology was as clear as the sky is blue, yet allopathic medicine knew only one way to react to his ailment: to surgically remove the gallstones. Though the procedure provided temporary and even life-saving relief, the approach also dismissed the underlying cause, which inevitably began searching for another suitable physical outlet. Anybody who has experienced the total removal of his or her gallbladder knows only too well how difficult it is to digest and assimilate any oily or fatty food from then on. Life just isn't the same after such a surgery.

To feel bitterness as an emotional disturbance can result in the physical symptom of feeling nauseous and vomiting of bitter vile bile. The emotional bitterness is causing the person to literally taste his acerbity.

If you want to learn more about the importance of your liver, I can recommend you read *The Healing Triad: Your Liver... Your Lifeline* by Dr. Jack Tips.

When the liver isn't happy anymore, it will finally dump the toxins into the KIDNEYS and BLADDER. The kidney's function centralizes on filtering out toxins from the blood and passing them out of the body via the urine. As the kidneys take on the extra load from the liver, they too can become overwhelmed and will now be susceptible to bacterial infections and kidney stones. The metaphysical aspect of the kidney speaks of experiencing fear, in particular about the future and finances. I have seen this phenomenon in my patients quite often where existential fear results in a kidney infection. Another aspect regarding the kidneys speaks of the relationship around our partnerships in love, business, and work in general. As the kidneys are comprised of two organs, the left and right kidneys, they symbolize a pair or a couple in relationship. This realm of partnership can be transferred and seen within us, where me meet our female and masculine side within one container, our integrated Self.

Core Body

Are you able to merge both aspects, feminine and masculine, within yourself in a harmonious way? Or are you entertaining this inner split and projecting externally onto your loved ones? Everybody we meet and with whom we engage in our lifetime ultimately represents a stark mirror reflecting the healing needs of our inner core wounds. Only by looking into the mirror can we truly find ourselves in our deepest core. We therefore have to seek out and locate what we are lacking in our outer world, even though what we search really lies within us all along.

Encounters with our partners are ultimately encounters with the unknown aspect of our inner self. Therefore, most of the difficulties, frustrations, and upsets we experience with our partners are basically the very challenges we face within ourselves. We generally do not like to look at this shadowy aspect as it feels uncomfortable and dark, and is often fear inducing. But only by embracing the true facts about ourselves can we truly engage in wholesome relationships with our loved ones and others. Once we start integrating these illuminated aspects into our consciousness we begin to see the real Self in another, now free of our projections.

The BLADDER is a wonderful and direct instrument in the way it expresses our unresolved emotions. Everyone can relate to how it feels to have a full bladder and how the increasing pressure forces us to release the urine as well as its pressure. A grieving or sad child, unable to cry during the day, might cry during the night, unconsciously shedding his tears in the form of bedwetting. Always look at the whole situation before you start scolding your child about soaked bed sheets!

In my clinical practice, mainly among women, I have observed reoccurring bladder infections, or cystitis, linked with a very distinct emotional set-up. The physical symptom of a cystitis attack results in a burning sensation before, during, or after urination, a truly painful experience! As the actual urine burns and stings on its release, so are the emotions of the inflicted person burning and stinging. A common scenario can be found in a married woman who feels deeply frustrated about her husband's behavior. Perhaps he doesn't show much interest in helping with the children or household chores. Initially, she may notice the

Core Body

imbalance and only feel a bit upset about it. Over time, however, such an emotionally energetic stagnation can culminate in deep resentment and frustration. After their lovemaking, she might feel the onset of her recurring cystitis due to the actual release of her suppressed emotions, even the negative ones, toward her husband. Remember, the second chakra is related to power, relationships, and honoring one another. As the woman continues to bury her anger and resentment deeply inside herself, they move more deeply into her womb and bladder. The internal emotional pressure, now withheld, builds up within her bladder and results in an acute or chronic infection. Again, with this infection we also see a bacterial component, yet the initial disturbance was created in the emotional realm.

Another example that explains this phenomenon is portrayed by the executive secretary of a high-powered corporate institution. Envision the following scenario: It is 4:30 p.m., the secretary has worked all day, in fact overtime, and is now really looking forward to her well-deserved evening. Suddenly her boss storms into her office, begging her to take care of the pile of work stacked up in his arms, work that needs to be completed for his presentation the following day. The woman's stomach sinks to the floor as she realizes once again that her evening will be taken over by tasks at work.

As this scenario played itself out last week and is now repeating itself, the woman feels angry, frustrated, and resentful. As she is dependent on the job and its high-paid salary she willingly takes care of her chores, yet deep inside she almost feels on the verge of an internal explosion. When week three comes around and this unacceptable work pattern continues, she feels the resurgence of sheer indignation and suppressed rage. Where does it all go? The secretary feels pissed off, angry, and enraged, and her external circumstances do not allow her to express what she really feels and thinks. If the weakest link in her body is her kidneys or bladder, the suppressed emotions will certainly manifest there as an initial bladder infection.

Whenever your next bladder infection appears ask yourself: *Who is pressurizing me? Which situation puts me under pressure? What do I need to let go of? Who or which situation makes me feel "pissed"?*

Core Body

When the kidneys cannot handle the toxins in the blood, the burden is passed on to the organ next in line, the LUNGS, as they deal with the expulsion of toxic gases. Here, we see symptoms like asthma and upper respiratory diseases, triggered by allergic processes. Have you ever considered that your halitosis (bad breath) might be linked to your toxic colon's expelling its putrid gases through your lungs? As the lungs feel overworked, their ability to exchange carbon dioxide and oxygen becomes more and more depleted, affecting the entire body, which is starving from its need for a vital oxygen supply.

Breathing requires two actions, inspiration and expiration. Every second of our life we breathe, and without breathing we would not be alive. Our breath is a clear indicator of our emotional realm in the way we say, "He takes my breath away," to describe a feeling of awe and wonder or possibly when we feel oppressed and limited by another's presence. This kind of fear and anxiety might also be expressed as: "I can't breathe, my chest is tight... I can't breathe."

We hear these expressions often from people suffering from asthma. In these cases, either the external or internal emotional frequencies are affecting the asthmatic in such a way as to interfere with his natural rhythm of breathing. An asthmatic can breathe in, but has severe problems breathing out. As with the toxic liver, the symptom of asthma is often created by several factors, such as chronic inflammation of the air passages. This makes the person with asthma highly sensitive to various triggers. And when the inflammation is stimulated by external and internal factors, the passages swell and fill with mucus. At this point the muscles within the breathing passages contract, causing further narrowing of the airways. This narrowing makes it difficult for the air to be breathed out, or exhaled, from the lungs, and the resistance to exhaling leads to the typical symptoms of an asthma attack.

Asthma is a prime example of the primary mechanism being damaged by cellular inflammation. Free radicals (molecules we do not want in our body) cause inflammation, and inflammation causes free radicals. Cellular inflammation is a severe terrain issue based on having too many toxins in the body. It is like having that garbage strike within your body, leaving you with piles and piles of accumulated trash.

Core Body

Usually the constantly alternating poles of inspiration and expiration create a smooth and uninterrupted rhythm. During meditation we become aware of the breath's pathways and where any congestion lies. Meditation's rhythmical up-and-down movement settles us into a relaxed position, allowing us to relate to life in a contemplative way, rather than rushing and reacting to our external world. The in-breath is dependent on the out-breath, as the out-breath is dependent on the in-breath. It is an interdependent marriage of two opposite poles unifying in one wholesome movement and enriching us with life. Often people with asthma experience an attack as a life-threatening suffocation. They fight for air and breathe in gasps with a throttled outbreath. In my practice, I see the intimate relationship of asthma to an intense underlying anxiety to almost everything that life has to offer. The person just can't relax, nor can he breathe out in a relaxed way and let go. Asthmatics tend to need to control their environment by having everything clean and sterile, and are often unable to joyfully experience the changing seasons of Nature, as the pollen count or environmental stimuli affect their overall breathing capacity.

Thorwald Dethlefsen and Rüdiger Dahlke agree: "asthmatics are afraid of life as life itself makes them afraid."

Whenever you experience your next asthma attack, ask yourself: *Which areas of life am I trying to avoid? What makes me anxious? What am I afraid of?*

From my years in clinical practice I feel it is important to strongly recommend not vaccinating any child with severe eczema or a history of asthma among the immediate family members. Today, through extensive clinical studies, we are aware of the direct relationship between skin eruptions like eczema and respiratory symptoms, particularly asthma. The skin and the lungs are indeed intimately related. For example, if there is a strong family history of asthma and a newborn suffers from a diaper rash or skin eruptions which were initially suppressed via externally applied cortisone or zinc creams, eventually the suppressed toxins will surely find their way into the child's next physical partner in line, the lungs. "Successfully" treating a child with asthma may eventually stimulate the still-dormant and suppressed eczema to rise to the surface again, which will be the signal to treat him or her with appropriate and indicated holistic treatments.

As the lungs cannot deal with the passing bucket, now filled with all kinds of toxins, it will be given to the body's general CIRCULATION system. We have two circulatory systems, the blood and the lymphatic system. The primary function of the lymph is to help detoxify the toxins in the blood. Yet, when the blood and lymphatic systems are overloaded, more waste is created by the poor cellular metabolism. Once the lymph system becomes congested, the whole body is affected, as the lymph cannot transport vital nutrients to each cell for its daily renewal. Now we are talking about a serious garbage pile-up! At that point, you can feel your swollen, painful lymph glands, at each side of the neck, under your armpits, in your groin, and/or anywhere else in the body.

And on we go. From the BLOOD and LYMPH SYSTEM the toxins continue to travel further to the SPLEEN and HEART. You can see the toxins are now affecting more and more of the interior of the body, attacking vital and life-preserving organs. The function of the spleen relies on filtering and cleansing the lymph, and thus serves as part of the body's waste disposal system. It is also intimately connected to our immune system. As the bloodstream is unable to pass the toxins to the already overloaded lymph, they will choose to travel to your heart. Dr. Jack Tips has said that "blood pressure can be a function of toxicity since the presence of toxins in the blood elevates blood pressure, as more fluid volume is required to buffer the toxins the kidneys can't handle."

If an individual also shows blood sugar imbalances, like insulin resistance, we can observe critical results due to the toxic onslaught affecting the heart muscle.

Needless to say, heart disease is the number-one killer in the U.S. today, next to colon cancer. Until 1930, heart attacks were rare, with only 3,000 occurring per year. By 1950, heart attacks increased to 500,000, and today in the U.S. people experience heart infarcts more than 1,255,000 times a year with an overall 200% increase. The number of U.S. citizens with diagnosed heart disease is 27 million and growing.

Many believe that conscious awareness originates in the brain alone—as if it is a separate entity from the body. Recent scientific research, however, suggests that consciousness actually emerges from the brain and the rest of the body acting together.

Our basic knowledge about the heart focuses around its function as a pump that circulates blood and generates pressure waves throughout the body. But the heart is much more than a muscular pump. It is an electromagnetic generator and an endocrine gland; it produces a wide range of electromagnetic frequencies; makes and releases numerous hormones; and is part of the central nervous system. Far more than a simple pump, scientists now recognize the heart as a highly complex system with its own functional brain. The human heart feels things the eyes cannot see and knows what the mind cannot understand.

Did you know that your heart beats 100,000 times a day, 40 million times a year, or some 3 billion times in the 70 to 80 years of a human life? Two gallons of blood per minute or 100 gallons an hour travel through your vessels and arteries with a combined length of 60,000 miles (more than twice the circumference of the Earth) through your body without your noticing this miraculous process at all. This all happens inside your body all the time!

Stephen Harrod Buhner, master herbalist and author of *The Secret Teachings of Plants* describes the heart in this way: "Little is known that the heart produces at least five different hormones (ANF, CNP, BNF, HPVD, CGRP), which have a broad impact on the organ, the brain, and body. These hormones strongly impact the hippocampus and integrated functions of the central nervous system that involves learning, memory, and exploratory activity in a new environment. The heart is directly wired into the central nervous system and brain and interconnected with all four brain centers."

We have all heard about the fascinating stories of the patient who, after receiving a heart transplant, suddenly craves different food articles or experiences not-his-own feelings, which appear instead to be tastes and sensations similar to those of the donor—and the donor's heart. The heart has its own memory!

Rollin McCraty, Ph.D., vice president and director of research at the Institute of HeartMath has informed us that research in the new discipline of neurocardiology shows that the heart is a sensory organ and a sophisticated center for receiving and processing information. The nervous system within the heart, or "heart brain," enables it to learn, remember, and make functional decisions independent of the brain's cerebral cortex. Moreover, numerous experiments have demonstrated that the signals the heart continuously sends to the brain influence the function of higher brain centers involved in perception, cognition, and emotional processing. It has been shown that information flowing through the human body impacts the brain only after the heart has first perceived it. How we perceive the world and our loved ones is determined by how our heart has received this information, before it sends it to the brain for further evaluation.

Our language speaks volumes when it comes to our heart. Expressions like "My heart was in my boots," or "Her heart leaped for joy," or "I have something on my heart," or "He takes things very much to heart" speak for themselves.

Heart symptoms force us to listen to our heart once again. High blood pressure symptoms can be a predisposing factor for a heart attack. Repressed aggression can be manifested in a blocked aggressive energy only to be released in a heart attack, meaning it is literally tearing the heart apart. The heart attack is then the result of all experienced attacks and beatings (whether physical or emotional) during the course of a lifetime, which the patient has ignored and left unresolved in the past.

My stepfather was a living example, suffering from multiple strokes over the span of 14 years. He suffered countless of heart attacks, from minor to severe, each time losing more of his mental and muscular capabilities. Louise Hay speaks of a heart attack as a suicide attempt that didn't come to reality or didn't work. Long before my stepfather actually left his body, his spirit had indicated its willingness to leave the world, as it was clear that deep inside himself he no longer enjoyed his stressful work life. His initial heart attacks were no more than small attempts to escape, yet ultimately left him spilt between two worlds simultaneously—the one where he wanted to live and the one where he longed to be on the other side.

Ask or tune into yourself and feel if your mind and heart are truly living in peaceful balance or if you are living a half-hearted life at this moment.

Core Body

In *Core Soul*, I will further explore this new paradigm of heart-centeredness, which serves as an integrated and vital ingredient in the changing of this New World, to guide you to live more from your heart and do so more deeply.

※

The heart not only deals with your unresolved emotions and external perceived frequencies, but also with your ever-growing pile of toxins. It may or may not be unable to meet its functional goals to keep you alive. In order to save your life, it will now dump the extra load onto your MUSCLES and SOFT TISSUE. Your aching body and muscles after a day of strenuous garden work might also be the result of your congested lymphatic system. When lactic acid builds up the muscles become stiff and sore, impacting your vertebrae and entire spine.

Rheumatism is an umbrella term for many symptoms that involve painfully shifting tissues that affect the joints and musculature. We all feel compassion when we see an elderly person riddled with rheumatism trying to lift himself out of his chair with all his mighty power. Overall stiffness makes moving an almost impossible task, yet as he slowly gets going the continued bodily movements seem to ease his overall stiffness and pain, at least for a while ... until he needs to rest once more. And the whole cycle starts again.

Such physical rigidity can also be seen in the mental sphere in a resistance to yield to life's ever-presenting changes. A clenching fist might symbolize withheld aggression or the desire to hit one's fist on the table. Here, repressed aggression inflames the joints and muscles, leaving them stiff and rigid. As the person softens his heart and mind and is willing to bend, he simultaneously allows his body and muscles to relax.

Continuing with our Toxic Stress Cycle, consistently constricted and spastic muscles now impact the SPINE, which impinges the nerve flow to various organs, which are then unable to effectively perform their functions.

As the toxic bucket is passed on, it is placed at the door of the BRAIN and NERVES. Now you are dealing with symptoms like Alzheimer's, dementia, and hyperactivity in children. The toxic levels of heavy metals or food allergies to food sensitivities are all part of this cycle. Food colorings, like Tartrazine, a synthetic lemon-yellow azo dye found in cheese and many other food articles, is known as a health-depleting toxin. Your ability or inability to think clearly during your workday might be the result of your body's having reached this stage within the unfolding Toxic Stress Cycle.

By now, with a weak heart and clogged brain, the overall communication within the body is significantly impaired and will eventually affect the ENDOCRINE GLANDS, whose function is based on hormone production. The master of the glandular system is called the hypothalamus, situated in the brain and regulating and communicating with all the other glands. These include the pituitary, pineal, thyroid, adrenal, pancreas, and testes or ovaries—just a few that make up this refined and very sensitive system. When the endocrine pathways of communication are interrupted as well, the next domino to fall is the DIGESTIVE SYSTEM. It is at this point that we may find it difficult to digest the meal on our plate because our enzymes are not doing the jobs they were meant to do.

So, here we are, having arrived full circle back at the top of our bodily scenic sightseeing tour! We are now looking at the very beginning of our daily plate and our digestive system, having addressed every major organ within the body by following the route of passing the bucket filled with overflowing toxins.

My sincere wish for you is that, after having read this chapter, you take the information and apply your attentive awareness to include the highest quality and best-selected foods in your diet. Doing so will not only feed but nourish you and help stabilize your entire body's functions by alleviating any detrimental effects that might affect you now and in the future.

Remember, your toxins are dancing through your body: from your digestive system to your colon; from your liver and gallbladder to your kidneys and bladder; from your lungs to your circulation with your blood and lymph; from your spleen and heart to your muscles and soft tissue;

Core Body

from your spine to your brain and nerves; from the brain and nerves to all your endocrine glands; and all the way back to your digestive system. It is one big toxic cycle!

The fact that we are still alive while we continue to bombard ourselves with unrecognizable and impossible-to-digest waste products, can only be contributed to our bodies' powerful intelligence, compassion, and magical ability to keep us that way.

How can we break this Toxic Stress Cycle? As already mentioned in our discussion about the Healing Triad of stomach, colon, and liver, any natural, holistic, and effective treatment based on the understanding of this principle is the first step to an overall physical healing. Once the source of toxicity is established and halted from traveling further throughout the body, an overall well-being and health can begin to resurface.

I can't stress enough here the value of the therapeutic tools of iridology and sclerology, as each person's iris and sclera clearly indicate the interrelationship between the stomach, colon, and liver.

Your conscious choice and your willingness to explore your relationship with your daily nutrition is ultimately the deciding denominator in your future health. To truly love your body, you have to eat healthy.

> I am not what happened to me. I am what I chose to become.
>
> —Carl Gustav Jung

The Essentials for Your Body to Move

> To be alive in this beautiful, self-organized universe,
> to participate in the dance of life with senses to perceive it,
> lungs that breathe it, organs that draw nourishment from it,
> it is a wonder beyond words.
>
> —Joanna Macy

It's time to eat! But this time, you don't just rush to the table or bite into a sandwich while trying to catch your next subway, calling this your breakfast. This time, you dance to your table, which offers you the most nurturing and delicious food. Your last visit to the beach inspired you to feel your body, allowing you to fall into yourself. Let's continue our walk on this golden inviting beach.

It is early morning and the air is filled with a slight crisp chill, slowly awakening the quiet and calm sea. The sand under your feet still feels cool, untouched by the rising sun. Noisy seagulls provide company in their search for their morning breakfast. A new day has risen, ready to embrace its unfolding life. As the fresh crisp air fills your lungs and body, you feel your inner mental and emotional freshness, too. It feels exquisitely pure, so in the here and now, so unmarred by negativity and external toxins that your sense of being alive is heightened. Your body becomes, and is, the new day!

Core Body

A table right on the beach, covered in white linen and decorated with color-bursting flowers and fresh life-giving food, is offered exclusively for your wellness. Your eyes skim over the bowls and plates filled with luminescent greens and fresh salad leaves and take in the rainbow of vibrant colors of the displayed exotic fruits. The intoxicating smell of their sun-kissed skins enriches your lungs with sheer delight. As you welcome the nurturing zest of freshly made meals, you become aware of how long it has been since you enjoyed being with your food. And while you drink a glass of fresh, clean water you notice the oxygenating sensation bubbling through all your cells, now ready to wake up. By taking time to look, taste, smell, and touch your food, other senses within you are gently awakening. You are distinctly aware that you only want to consume food that will not taint or squash your already embodied vitality. In fact, this morning you want to touch, smell, and taste the same alive resonance and vibrancy manifested through food that you already feel inside yourself. As you honor yourself you honor the food in front of you, reminding you to swirl around your body and lift your arms high up into the blue sky....

You are ready to greet this day with your morning dance and a smile.

Whenever my parents mentioned the subject of food or gathered around the family table to enjoy their meal, my body responded with confusion and a sense of heaviness. There were days I really was hungry and I wanted to eat, and then there were all the other days when I was painfully reminded of my physical limitations regarding food. Being born with the incapacity to digest proteins resulting in the mal-absorption of nutrients, and hence a complete vegetarian, I was left with only a handful of food choices. I grew up mainly on pasta and salads, avoiding meat, fish, and the rich German diet. Emotional tension and general nervousness also affected my entire digestive system, and years of intestinal ailments followed. I wasn't anorexic or bulimic, yet whatever I ate clearly didn't respond to or correspond with my body. The idea of eating became a virtual nightmare!

Core Body

Over the years, I tried all different approaches to finding the right diet, from macrobiotic and vegan to liquid and raw food. I took an arsenal of supplements hoping to heal my intestines, and interfaced them with some juice fasting. As I was personally afflicted, I know very well how frustrating it can be to be constantly on the lookout, having to choose the right and least disturbing food articles. Going to a restaurant became a waste of time, scanning the menu up and down to try to find any suitable dishes. By now I had developed gluten sensitivity with diverticulitis, a spastic colon, and chronic intestinal inflammation. Anything, even a spoon of rice, could make me curl up with abdominal pain. There were days I stopped eating altogether just to calm the pain, which returned immediately after I ate some food again. It was another vicious cycle!

As I started to heal mentally, emotionally, and physically, I realized that most diet plans on the market today still focus on the isolated parts of human health rather than work with the whole nutritional picture. Somehow, my primal instinct, my gut feeling, was telling me that the idea of a healthy nutrition had to be based on simple nutritional building blocks rather than another therapy. I knew simplicity with a sense of ease would eventually change the food crisis in my body.

Food, as a nutritional energy provider, is such an essential part of our lives and existence. Every day we are given the choice to build and support our health through nutrition as well as manifest our future health. Sometimes patients walk into my office carrying full shopping bags filled with their latest vitamins and mineral supplements. Their breakfast looks more like a handful of pills and capsules to be swallowed with their favorite smoothie and a run around the block. There is nothing wrong with a delicious morning smoothie. But often people rely on the external substitution of supplements rather than fundamental life-sustaining nutrition. Some of my patients have jumped from one detoxification program to the next, cleansing the body to excess without taking time to rebuild the body. Strong and lasting health can only be created with a nutritional plan that resonates with Nature's Law; anything else culminates in superficial attempts. Eating or following a diet plan should not be a therapy; nor should it place overall restrictions on the person already ailing with digestive symptoms. Instead it should be inviting and of a flexible and varied nature. As you become an ambassador for your body and health, you will want your food to be fresh, organic, vibrant, and alive, with no questions asked.

With 67% of Americans currently obese or overweight, 27% with high blood pressure, and a whopping 96% who cannot recall the last time they had a salad or a serving of fresh vegetables, it is no wonder that this country, and the world, is so sick. Most diseases today are in fact caused by a poor diet. Throughout this book, you will read about the fascinating discovery that the environment in which we live and which lives in us directly affects our cellular behavior. This phenomenon clearly speaks the same language when we talk about nutrition. What and when we eat is a major factor in determining our biochemical terrain. A faulty and inadequate diet stresses our gastrointestinal lining with mucosa; inhibits the function of the liver; taxes the kidneys; and damages the heart and brain along with our immune system. The display of food on your plate affects your entire body!

Today, nutritional researchers estimate that 90% of our diseases are caused or aggravated by improper food consumption, causing nutritional deficiencies and excesses with autointoxication or low oxygen. Further, fermentation in the bowel poisons the blood and lymph, resulting in poor elimination of toxins and metabolic wastes. All three of these causes are nutritional issues.

As our lifestyle is very much removed from the idyllic surroundings of clean fresh air and rich soils, we need to have a closer look at how we can meet our physical needs within our present and challenging environment. Most of the population, particularly in cities, spend their weekdays in office buildings padded with insulation to save energy costs, lined with toxic carpets and wall paints, sitting under artificial lights, and eating over-cooked canteen food, all of which add to the general lack of oxygen supply to the cells. During the lunch break, a quick escape to the nearest green park won't fill this void either, as we now breathe in air polluted by the combustion of cars and surrounding industrial fumes. Daily work stress and/or personal emotional stress keeps adding to the cellular lack of oxygen supply, as well as our poor diet, which again causes a lack of oxygen as well as a drained energy reservoir in the body. From the quick cup of coffee, carbonated drink, donuts, and deli sandwiches to the alcohol consumption after work, we are consuming huge amounts of acidic products, all of which contribute to our cells being starved of the oxygen they need to produce energy. Without energy our cells die prematurely. Premature cell death means we get sick and age at a faster rate.

Once there is less oxygen supply available for the general metabolism, lactic acid starts to build up and changes the cellular environment to a more acidic terrain, resulting in the degeneration and destruction of cells. A low oxygen supply within the body is the fundamental baseline for the creation of any illness. Therefore, a fresh and healthy diet, as well as clean, fresh and oxygen-rich water, is a vital ingredient regarding the oxygen supply to our cells and tissues.

The best nutrition is based on its well-functioning biochemistry and bioenergy. Our food not only affects our cellular biochemistry, but also deeply impacts our energetic matrix and bioenergy, the vital force within our bodies. A well-balanced diet creates a peaceful equilibrium in the mind, body, and soul by stimulating our inherent highest intelligence to heal itself. Diet influences state of mind, and state of mind influences the choice of diet. You might also say that good nutrition is an expression of our state of "beingness" and of our harmony with the universal laws of creation. In this way, your food becomes your medicine.

Let's have a look at the four essential building blocks of food, and how we can create a healthy and nutritional diet.

VEGETABLES AND FRUITS

As I started to heal, my body craved and preferred more and more vibrant and alive food. If I didn't have some "living food" on my plate, I felt an immediate physical response. I am not a die-hard raw food follower, but a huge percentage of my food now consists of fresh, raw, and organically grown vegetables and fruits. I just love it and so does my body! Each time I look at the luminous orange color of my carrot soup, I literally feel the energy of the sun and the minerals of the Earth running right through my body. Our bodies need and thrive on fresh vegetables and fruits. I am sometimes asked if I would prefer a complete raw food diet. Personally, I prefer diversity, which includes the freedom to play and explore with food. Lightly cooked vegetables provide an inner cell factor, called chromatin, which is rich in DNA and RNA, vital and important building blocks within the body. These essential factors are either unavailable, or supplied within a minimum range, if the person chooses strictly a full raw food diet. Raw food in itself is encased in indigestible cellulose, which can only be broken down by a very light steaming or cooking process. It is best to always consume a variety of raw and lightly steamed vegetables next to your protein meal as, in this way, you are provided a wide spectrum of enzymes and easily digestible nutrients at the same time.

Proteins are a real challenge for the body, as they are initially toxic and need to be detoxified first by the liver. Vegetables provide a wonderful enzyme-rich spectrum and are essential in assisting the body with the entire process of protein assimilation and elimination. It might sound simple, but fresh, organic vegetables serve as your future prevention of diseases such as colon cancer, reabsorption of bowel gases, and prostate problems. Raw vegetables provide an immediate enzyme supply that helps properly digest proteins and the fiber and roughage to disperse these proteins. Further, the enzymes from raw vegetables aid in the protein's transformation to amino acids. Proteins cannot function within the body unless they are broken down into amino acids. How about starting your day with a health-promoting raw vegetable juice, created with a variety of organically grown vegetables or fruits? I say, bring it on!

In *Raw Food, Real World*, top New York chef and restaurateur Matthew Kenney and his partner Sarma Melngailis state: "The more you eat raw foods, the more your body starts to crave them over anything else."

In 1930, Paul Kouchakoff, M.D. presented a paper at the First International Congress of Microbiology titled "The Influence of Food Cooking on the Blood Formula of Man." In it, Dr. Kouchakoff reported that eating a live-food diet did not produce leukocytosis, or an unhealthy number of white blood cells. When foods are cooked on the other hand, the resultant energy fields are not able to resonate immediately with the body and actually respond more with a defensive nature.

If the food we eat is too hot, it can actually disrupt the enzyme system in the gastric mucosa as well as injure the gastric mucus linings. The other extreme occurs when we consume iced drinks and too-cold foods that slow down the enzyme function and peristalsis action within the colon. Most researchers indicate that overall nutrient destruction, or loss of bioavailability, after cooking is an approximate but staggering 85%!

Fresh and wholesome food carries a stronger frequency and radiance as seen in the photographs done with Kirlian photography, photographic techniques used to capture the phenomenon of electrical discharge. Researchers have found that a luminescent field, like a naturally colored radiation, surrounds food articles. Kirlian photography has clearly demonstrated that live food emanates a much stronger auric and luminescent field than heated, cooked, or even microwaved food. As we consume this adulterated food, now with far less radiance, we are lowering our life force to a less potent frequency. All living organisms are made of patterns of resonant energy, or organizing fields, which interplay and interact with each other, from human to animal to the plant kingdom.

As our environment influences the behavior of our cells, we cannot ignore the fact anymore that what we eat, how much stress we have, and how we live all directly affect our gene expression. Yet, remember, you are not a victim of your genes and inherited blueprint. Through proper living, a wholesome diet, a balanced lifestyle, exercise, and a mental, emotional, and spiritual harmonious relationship to life, you have the opportunity to activate your genes to function in accordance with your highest quality of well-being. Your attentive harmony with your food and drink brings you closer to Nature's design.

Simply, you are what you eat! Every 28 days, your skin replaces itself and every five months your liver gives birth to a complete new generation of liver cells. Your bones go through this cycle every 10 years. Your body makes new cells from the very food you eat. What you eat literally becomes you! Why not reclaim your choice about what you're made of?

Core Body

In the *Essene Gospel of Peace, Book One* by Szekeley, Jesus is quoted as saying: "For I tell you truly, live only by the fire of life, and prepare not your foods with the fire of death, which kills your foods, your bodies and your souls also."

PROTEINS

Proteins are the main building blocks of all life, and therefore vitally important at every level. Your immune system's antibodies, your hormones, your extra-cellular matrix (the material between the cells), your collagen (the cement that holds the cells together), your bones, and teeth, your brain's neurotransmitters, and all your enzymes are made from protein or organized components of proteins, called amino acids. The body's vital amino acids are derived primarily from our daily diet. As soon as the proteins are consumed the body's processes convert them into amino acids. Here, the liver is of utmost importance, as it "humanizes" dietary proteins into usable amino acids. It is like giving the amino acid with no name an identity. This allows the amino acid to recognize its function and purpose within your body. From being a non-self, it now lives as its self. Without this vital function of the liver, proteins, or converted amino acids, would remain foreign and unusable in the body. What happens when the liver is unable to humanize the proteins? They move around the body as foreign invaders without name, identity, or passport. This causes the immune system to wake up, realizing it must attack these strangers. This is the very reason for such events like your yearly seasonal allergy episodes, in which the immune system is attacking the unrecognized foreigners in your body.

In general, the body "reads" the proteins in fruit, vegetables, meat, viruses, bacteria, and parasites, as well as airborne pollens the same way—as non-distinctive information—because all these substances have essentially the same makeup. This is the reason we need the liver to examine and eliminate each incoming protein for its importance and usability. As the immune system is now on alert to fight the unrecognized invaders, the body expresses this internal battle as a seasonal allergy attack. It is actually a weakened left liver lobe, and not only the surrounding pollens flying around you, that is causing your sneezing fits, watery eyes, and dripping nose.

Did you know that food allergies and sensitivities are some of the most commonly miss- and undiagnosed medical conditions in the U.S.? An estimated 10 to 30% of the population suffers from this illness triggered by environmental causes. Food allergies and sensitivities annually result in countless lost workdays at an estimated cost of $500 million a year (Journal of Allergy and Clinical Immunology). Did you also know that a weak liver and digestive system primarily, although not exclusively, causes the dreaded morning sickness in pregnant women? Remember, excess proteins can putrefy the colon, which affects the whole immune system, pH levels in the blood, and overloads the lymphatic system.

I hope you now appreciate what a healthy meal should look like. Your nutritional pyramid consists of fresh vegetables, some necessary proteins, followed by high quality oils and complex carbohydrates with plenty of fresh fruits, preferably grown in their local environment. I highly recommend introducing fermented foods to your diet as well, such as sauerkraut. Fermented foods improve the digestion, restore the proper balance of bacteria in the gut, are rich in enzymes, increase vitamin content, and help us absorb the nutrients we consume.

Our late morning and lunch meal should include about 65 to 75% of a variety of at least five different vegetables or a salad with a small portion of 25 to 30% protein at one meal. Today, most people eat an incorrect amount of protein. Mostly the ratio leans to too much, rather than too little. In terms of metabolic combustion, excess protein in the diet does not burn cleanly. In fact, it creates an over-acid terrain due to the accumulation of the body's own created waste by-products. This opens the door for symptoms of arthritis, kidney damage, schizophrenia, osteoporosis, atherosclerosis, heart disease, and cancer. Experts around the world suggest that the most sufficient protein requirement is around 25 to 35 grams per day; less if the protein we eat comes from live foods. It is interesting to note that the average protein concentration in mother's milk is just 1.4%, perfectly sufficient to supply the human organism with all the essential amino acids and proteins needed during a time of most-demanded growth.

Core Body

We all assimilate our proteins differently. Those of us who are genetically fast oxidizers—who metabolize the proteins faster—need a higher amount of protein. Others are genetically slow oxidizers who produce their biochemical energy best on a meal with less protein. As mentioned, no one diet exists for all, as each of us is a unique individual with individual needs.

The controversial issue of whether vegetarians receive enough proteins in their diet has created unfounded fear and countless theories. It is true that incomplete amino acid structures are taken over by the small intestines before they are ready for absorption in order to complete the process. When this happens, the lymphatic system can become congested with large molecular proteins from complex vegetable sources, like unfermented soybeans, raw nuts, peanuts, and so on. Yet, according to the Max Planck Institute for Nutritional Research in Germany, considered to be the most respected and reliable nutritional research organization in the world, there are many vegetable sources of protein that are superior or equal to animal proteins. The Max Planck Institute has found that complete vegetarian proteins, which contain all eight essential amino acids, to be available in almonds, sesame, pumpkin, and sunflower seeds, buckwheat, all leafy greens, and most fruits. Fruits supply approximately the same percentage of complete protein as mother's milk. And if the protein is taken in its live-food form, even less is needed.

As I was born a natural vegetarian, I do take a supplement with my main meals, which provides all essential amino acids and peptide chains. The supplement not only enhances and completes my protein structure, but also allows my body to assimilate up to three times more protein without the added fats and carbohydrates. It therefore preserves my lymphatic nucleoprotein pool, essential to all my healthy bodily functions. This means that although I do not consume meat or fish, my body is still nurtured by all the necessary proteins.

In *Spiritual Nutrition* Gabriel Cousens points out: "As our system changes with meditation, fasting, eating lighter, and increasing live-food intake, our cell membranes become clear, more porous and thinner, so the protein we take in moves into the cells more readily. With reduced blockage, more of the protein we eat pushes itself through the cell membrane into the cells, so our protein needs spontaneously drop."

It is important to mention here that vegans and live-food lovers of all ages do show a tendency for vitamin B12 deficiency. Research has shown that 80% of the vegan and live-food population display a disposition for sub-clinical or clinical B12 deficiency with increased homocysteine levels within 6 to 10 years, a condition which plays a role in destroying the lining of the artery walls, promotes the formation of blood clots, and accelerates the buildup of scar tissue. This event can be particular damaging in newborn babies whose vegetarian mothers didn't add extra vitamin B12 into their diet or supplement protocols. A lack of vitamin B12 in the mother's diet can contribute to a severe lack of myelin in nerve tissues and subsequent neurological developments. It is vital, therefore, that any vegan and pregnant mother supplement with vitamin B12 during her pregnancy and breastfeeding period and eat plenty of sea vegetables and spirulina to meet this deficiency.

Proteins provide us with strength and stamina, whereas carbohydrates provide us with energy. In brief summary, eating too much protein or too little protein can cause problems, as follows:

Excessive protein consumption can result in osteoporosis, teeth and gum diseases, high cholesterol, acidity in the body, constipation, a toxic lymphatic system, kidney infection and weakness, a swollen, over-oxidized liver, water retention, chronic degenerative diseases like arthritis, diabetes, cancer, allergies, hypertension, and a poor immune response.

Protein deficiencies can result in glandular fatigue like adrenal burnout and anemia, the inability to use amino acids for metabolic processes, a weakened immune system, stringy muscles, degenerative diseases, an inability to heal, a slow metabolism with symptoms like cold hands and feet or weight gain, an accelerated aging processes, hair loss, depression, memory loss, deep fatigue, infertility, alkalosis, and low blood sugar.

The first rule of a good digestion and assimilation of protein is based on the fundamental principle of not mixing major portions of protein and carbohydrates/starch at the same time. Dr. A. Stuart Wheelwright states clearly that eating proteins with carbohydrates is a major cause of elevated cholesterol within the body.

Why are so many people allergic to cow's milk today? Well, milk is a combined product of proteins and carbohydrates, or sugars. As soon as proteins and carbohydrates are separated within the diet plan, environmental and food allergies are drastically ameliorated. Your seasonal watery and itching eyes are directly linked to your plate! If we truly start to become aware of our inner responses to food we may be able to avoid food allergies all together.

THE BEST QUALITY OILS

Before the body can use any protein it has to be made nontoxic by the liver. This process adds a little bit of unsaturated fat to the protein molecule. As your digestion is connected to and interconnected with proteins, carbohydrates, and oils, it is therefore important to choose the best high-quality oils for your diet plan. Don't save money here; buy the best! The body requires both saturated and unsaturated fats for its life purposes. What do saturated and unsaturated fats mean to your diet and health? These terms describe how many hydrogen atoms occur in a molecule, or fundamental unit, of fats and oils as compared to carbon atoms. A fatty acid molecule is one of the building block of fat, and the more hydrogen than carbon that it has, the more saturated it is. Saturated fats are usually solid at room temperature (think of bacon grease or a block of cheese). The fewer hydrogen atoms to carbon atoms, the more liquid the fat is (think of canola or sunflower seed oil).

To maintain optimal health, the oils we eat should mainly come from seeds and vegetables. These essential fatty acids are critical when it comes to a well-functioning brain and heart. In my practice I suggest high doses of selected ratios of omega-3, -6, and -9 oils for all my autistic children. These children are in need of good oils and very much thrive on them. Have you ever seen an autistic child literally dip his finger in a lump of butter? This is to let us know that his body craves this valuable fat.

Core Body

Optimal fat contribution is another prime essential for the body to live and dance in optimal health. Always remember to use the best high-quality oils for your protein and vegetable meals. Today, bad oils and excess sugar cause most diseases. Bad oils are the major cause of cancer, hardened arteries, high blood pressure, heart attacks, low blood sugar, obesity, food sensitivities, sluggish liver, gallstones, hormonal imbalances, and allergies. The cheap supermarket cooking oils destroy most of the nutritive fats like omega-3 fats, creating carcinogenic and mutagenic by-products. And yes, I am talking here about your McDonald's cheeseburger with those added fries.

Did you know that your bag of potato chips can contain up to 500 times more acrylamide (a naturally occurring chemical compound found in many plant-based, high-carbohydrate foods after they are heated) than is allowed in drinking water by the World Health Organization? This natural chemical in high doses can cause both benign and malignant stomach tumors, and due damage to the central and peripheral nervous system.

Oils are comprised of a fatty acid, called Vitamin F, which is actually an essential nutrient present in raw or soaked nuts, whole grains, beans, avocado, and seeds, especially flax seed. This vitamin is very important for the thyroid and adrenal glands, nerve sheaths (so important in people suffering from multiple sclerosis), hair, skin, and all mucus membranes. Good oils, like omega-3 oil, balance elevated cholesterol, whereas bad oils increase it. The good oils, known as EPA and DHA, are most commonly found in fish, flax, and pumpkin seed oil, and are wonderful beneficial fats for the body.

The very best fatty acid is oleic acid, commonly found in extra-virgin cold-pressed organic olive oil, as it protects the heart and reduces cholesterol. All these fine essential fatty acids regulate cholesterol and bad triglycerides, as well as nurture and repair our cell membranes. A strong and healthy cell membrane keeps you healthy and younger.

Oils are also very important when it comes to inflammatory symptoms accompanied with swelling, redness, and heat. Most polyunsaturated fats, which spoil more quickly than saturated fats, even when you store them in the refrigerator, such as safflower, sunflower, corn, peanut, and soy, are high in linoleic acid, an omega-6 essential fatty acid that the body converts into arachidonic acid, and some prostaglandins, which all have a predominantly pro-inflammatory influence on the body. These oils contain almost no omega-3, so essential for soothing inflammation. To function well via a balanced and healthy body you not only need high-quality oils, but a balanced ratio of omega -3, -6, -9 oils.

Our prehistoric ancestors ate mainly a diet with a ratio of omega-6 to omega-3 ratio of 1:1. Today, the current ratio is anywhere between 10:1 and 25:1. Products with a ratio of 4:1 are excellent, especially in brain conditions. Start introducing into your diet your daily doses of flax-seed oil or borage oil next to your daily fish oil and your body will become your "smooth operator."

You can also incorporate the best olive oil or flax seed oil for optimal use, followed by grape seed oil or unrefined sesame oil for your favorite salads. Green olive oil, used once a week, can be helpful in the prevention of gallstones. Coconut oil is another great oil—just watch for rancidity—along with hemp seed and macadamia oil.

COMPLEX CARBOHYDRATES

Proteins build our daily foundation, whereas carbohydrates give us the basic fuel for energy. Today, most people over-consume bad carbohydrates and lack high-quality carbohydrates. Did you know that carbohydrates include all starches and sugars like alcohol, squash, bubble gum, and pasta and apple pie? Carbohydrates, the sugar elements that fuel us with energy, are literally everywhere. Complex carbohydrates are starches in their most natural states, like potatoes, starchy vegetables, and legumes. "Complex" means they can't be digested easily and require several steps for their completion process. This slower process is necessary so the precious energy supply isn't wasted too quickly. When we talk about refined carbohydrates, we are talking about donuts, soda, and the typical junk food diet of the average American. This diet produces too far too much fast-burning fuel, leaving us stressed and literally burnt out. Why not add some sesame seeds for your next snack, which have three times the carbohydrate content of red cabbage, mung bean sprouts, green snap beans, and many other fruits and vegetables?

Most refined carbohydrates also have lost their silicon component. Today, we know that emotional disorders associated with a lack of silicon include schizophrenia and neurosis. A silicon deficiency is also associated with a desire for tobacco and with substance abuse.

Most people eat a high-carbohydrate and low-protein diet, the culprit of many inflammatory symptoms within the body. Research has shown that a low-carbohydrate diet in women significantly reduces cellular and tissue inflammation. Always remember, we fall ill with the consumption of sugar and bad fats!

And another note: Do not drink liquids with your meal, particularly when you eat proteins. Your stomach produces hydrochloric acid, which is needed to digest the proteins, yet becomes too diluted if you drink while you eat. If you experience chronic yeast infections or candida this is important, as the hydrochloric acid protects your body against bacteria and yeast entering the small intestines, the next step in the digestive process.

I am not a keen follower of diet books, as often they do not understand the importance of cellular healing in combination with the circadian rhythm, or correct timing of eating (more about this in the next chapter). Therefore, I highly recommend the book THE PRO-VITA! PLAN: Your Foundation For Optimal Nutrition by Dr. Jack Tips (available at www.appleadaypress.com) as it addresses these vital issues. The Pro-Vita! Plan not only nourishes health at the cellular level, but also strengthens the body in its ability to digest its given food once again. Painful digestive disorders, from irritable bowel syndrome, spastic colon, ulcerative colitis, and Crohn's disease to celiac and gluten sensitivity disorders can all be balanced and healed again. Eating food should be fun and a total delicious experience, rather than something unbearable to face each and every day. I am the walking testimonial here!

To create a diet for ourselves requires mindfulness and purpose with a fundamental understanding why we eat certain foods and what we want from our diet. A wholesome nutrition not only keeps you healthy

Core Body

and vibrant, but also facilitates the assimilation, storage, conduct, and transmission of the cosmic and evolutionary energies, which we all need now to create this New World. With 34 million adult Americans considered obese, there is some real concern for the spiritual state of this country. In contrast, a synthesis of your breath, sunlight, the direct cosmic energy that pours through your crown chakra, the nurturing electromagnetic energy coming from the Earth, and vital, wholesome food you can sustain yourself in the most vibrant and highest form of living. To live and be authentic requires authentic food!

Gabriel Cousens, M.D. in Conscious Eating eloquently states: "Our food choices reflect the ongoing harmony with ourselves, the world, all of creation, and the Divine."

Next time you go shopping, buy some soul food!

֍

You danced well this time! Imagine how light and effortless your next dance will be with a body nurtured with alive and fresh food. Then go further. Envision how your mental clarity and mindfulness is joining the movement of your body and soul to result in a dance fueled by your unlimited and ever-present creativity. Your life and dance is getting better and better....

Dance is the fastest, most direct route to the truth.
—Gabrielle Roth

The Natural Timing of Your Dance

When attention and presence become one,
the world that is moving outside takes on the fragrance of that unity.

—Mooji

You attend a beautiful ballet performance at the theater. The lights start to dim, the heavy maroon velvet curtains rise slowly toward the ceiling to reveal the decorated stage, and for a brief moment, the theater enthralls its audience again with its timeless magic. The music starts with an overwhelming entry of violins, horns, percussion, and flutes. From each side of the stage, one by one, the ballerinas arrive, filling the performance space in total synchronicity. As none steps out of line, you watch with awe this choreographed unity, which slowly becomes an emotional and individual experience for each of the spectators in the theater. The exact moment of movements and timing is perfect, practiced diligently to the minute details. The arms, the gesture of the dancers' hands to the position of their fingers, all is in unison with the surrounding music. Nobody takes the lead, nobody steps out of line, and nobody dominates the space. Each one of these dancers knows his and her position and moves with exact timing to be part of this unified performance. The sheer fact that each dancer is able to acutely listen and respond to the timing of the conductor as he is leading his orchestra, and at the same time merges with the group dynamic of the other dancers is a testimonial to the art in movement. We, the spectators, are in awe and mesmerized by these seemingly effortless swirling bodies, entrancing us with their elegance and grace.

Within our body lies an inner clock, a natural rhythm that influences numerous physical functions. It is called the circadian rhythm, representing the roughly 24-hour cycle in the physiological processes of living beings, including plants, animals, fungi, and cyanobacteria. In a strict sense, circadian rhythms are endogenously (built-in or self-sustaining) generated, although they can be modulated by external cues such as sunlight and temperature. Circadian rhythms are important in determining the sleeping and feeding patterns of all animals, including human beings. There are clear patterns of brain wave activity, hormone production, cell regeneration, and other biological activities linked to this daily cycle. We all are keenly aware that our circadian rhythm is interrupted when we experience jet lag that stretches over a few days after the arrival of an international flight, for example, when we feel our stomach start growling at 3:00 a.m. According to our built-in clock it is lunchtime! Today, the concept of circadian rhythm is often overlooked or mentioned as one individual aspect of the daily cycle, yet rarely incorporated within our personal rhythms of the day.

Time Magazine (December 2009) published an article titled "The Sorry State of American Health" in which it stated: "Despite advances in medicine, Americans are less healthy than we used to be, and the next generation may be worse off. In spite of our gleaming hospitals and cutting-edge technology, on some basic health measures the U.S. is starting to fall behind—far behind."

The U.S. spends far more on health care than any other nation in the world. Yet despite the high expenditure, the country is not healthier, and shows staggering statistics of a higher infant-mortality rate and shorter lifespans than many other developed nations. Not only is this a dangerous way to practice medicine, but it is also a breathtakingly expensive one. In 2005, Americans paid out a record of $2 trillion on health care with a projected spending in 2020 of $4,64 trillion, making it the world's top spender on things that should clearly be prolonging and enhancing their lives. Due to the lack of a basic wellness-infrastructure, however, today nearly 1.5 million people experience a new or recurrent heart attack each year. Just take a moment and think about this fact! Approximately one-third of these attacks are recurrent.

The American Cancer Society estimates that in 2013 about 102,480 people will be diagnosed with colorectal cancer, which is the third leading cause of death in the U.S. with about 50,830 deaths. Thousands of deaths each year could have been avoided with timely and effective health care.

The biggest problem in the U.S. healthcare system, as well as in that of many other developed countries, is that it has been strongly designed to respond to illness rather than its prevention at the expense of the totality of the whole person.

As this book speaks of core aspects within us, the Core Mind, the Core Body, and the Core Soul, let's have a look at the most simplest and most fundamental building-blocks within the body that profoundly serve us in the prevention of future illness.

❧

As you gather more information, you will learn the core principles behind all physical and biochemical imbalances in the body. In my view, these important chapters regarding our circadian rhythms and pH analysis (the scale measurement of how acidic, or basic, a substance is) should be included in any standard medical curriculum and training, whether allopathic or alternative. If everybody followed these basic rules of natural timing designed by Nature itself, we would not only establish a platform of health that acts as a preventative measure for our future well-being, but would also be able to reduce the overwhelming number of stories of chronic and degenerative diseases. Remember, it all starts and ends on your plate!

First I will describe the following concept of circadian rhythms in very simple terms. I am sure by the end of this section, you will get the idea.

In Chinese acupuncture, the meridian clock is a 24-hour cycle that portrays the body's complete functions and its relationship with diet.

For example, the large intestines begin to function at about 5 to 7 a.m., followed by the stomach at 7 to 9 a.m., when we generally consume our breakfast. Then at 9 to 11 a.m. the pancreas continues the digestive process, and so on. Every two hours, day and night, another organ takes over the entire metabolism of the body. Isn't that a marvelous invention?

These natural cycles are just like the ebb and tide of our oceans or the monthly cycles of new and full moon. They happen of their own accord, yet impact us profoundly on the mental, emotional, and physical levels. Knowing about such natural cycles makes it easier for us to adapt our lifestyle and eating habits. As we focus on the nutritional aspect, we can see how this rhythm influences the acid and alkaline pH levels in the body.

The pH balance of the human bloodstream is one of the most important biochemical mechanisms in the human body. The body actually deposits and withdraws minerals from within in order to maintain a proper level. A balanced pH, a measure of the concentration of the hydrogen ion, is also required to achieve good health, improve immunity, maintain good sleep patterns, energy levels, a healthy weight, appetite, and food desires, and regulate perspiration and our mental state. Symptoms like tingling in the extremities, headaches, cold hands and feet, strong smelling urine, and aches and pains are all expressions of an imbalanced pH level. The more imbalanced pH levels are, the more the individual is likely to develop health problems or struggle with his weight. Additionally, feeling tired, lethargic or generally unwell are also symptoms of an imbalanced pH level. If a person stays too long in an acid state, symptoms like rheumatoid arthritis, diabetes, lupus, tuberculosis, osteoporosis, and cancer can occur. All inflammatory conditions can be related to an elevated acidic state. On the other hand, if the person stays too long in the alkaline, or opposite, state, there can be manifestations of constipation, flu, heart trouble, indigestion, and bacterial and viral infections.

pH functions have a profound impact on our mental and emotional states, too. For example, if you are too acidic, you might experience anxiety, extroverted behavior, nervousness, or hyperactivity with rapid heartbeats. Conversely, if you are too alkaline, then you are prone to general sluggishness and introverted behavior with fatigue in the morning. When the whole system is sluggish, the digestive system is affected with indigestion and overall fermentation. I feel strongly that if one's imbalanced pH level were acknowledged and treated, mental imbalances like depression, bipolar disorder, anxiety, panic attacks and as psychotic states could greatly alleviated without the commonly prescribed anti-psychotic and anti-depressant medications.

The term pH stands for potential hydrogen. Its levels control the speed of the body's biochemical reactions. When the pH is too acid our body's chemical reactions and electrical actions are too fast, leaving us burnt out and stressed. On the other hand, when the pH is too alkaline, all our processes are too slow, resulting in autointoxication, or self-poisoning. The presenting and related ailments then have a sluggish and congested nature.

The pH scale goes from 0 to 14; a pH of 7.0 is therefore neutral. Please note that the pH is a dynamic state of ebb and flow and should not be seen as a linear condition. For general purposes, however, any value above or below 7.0 is considered either alkaline or acid. For example, if we apply the pH scale to our nutrition, 0 to 7.0 represents acidic foods and 7.1 to 14 represents alkaline foods.

All foods are classified as alkalizing or acidifying based on the effect the food has on urine pH after consumption. If a food increases the acidity of urine after consumption, it is classified as an acidic food; if a food increases the alkalinity of urine after consumption, it is classified as an alkalizing food. Most vegetables are examples of alkalizing foods and all meats are examples of acidic foods. The body tries to maintain an alkalizing pH of 7.35 to 7.45, with 7.4 being the general average. As our continuously changing bodies and environments demand different requirements today, Dr. A. Stuart Wheelwright and many other authorities agree on a slightly changed pH optimal range as 5.8 to 6.8, rather than the textbook number of 7.4.

The common pH test procedures are via the urine or saliva, each fluid providing specific results. The optimal reading for the urine is 5.8 to 6.8 with slight variances for climate, and for the saliva 6.4 to 6.8. After eating, the saliva pH should rise to 7.8 or higher. If you are interested in testing your urine and saliva pH levels, test tapes, available over-the-counter, can be purchased at any health food shop or pharmacy.

One of the most important functions governed by the pH is the reaction of our enzymes and how fast, slow, or effectively we burn our fuel or energy to stay alive. Enzymes are energized protein molecules necessary for life. They catalyze and regulate nearly all biochemical reactions that occur within the human body. Enzymes turn the food we eat into energy and unlock this energy for use in the body. They cannot be seen with even the most powerful microscope, but improved blood and immune system functioning can determine their presence and strength. We naturally produce both digestive and metabolic enzymes as they are needed, and any surplus can be stored by the organs for later use or used as fuel for the brain. The enzymes, which digest our food, can only function within a certain range of pH level. For example, the enzyme pepsin in the stomach can only be active in an acid environment, one that is not higher than the number 5 on our scale, and the steak (or any meat) on your plate requires an acid environment to be well digested. With an out-of-range pH, the body is unable to assimilate nutrients, vitamins, or minerals. This means you may feel as if you are enjoying your food, but its nutrients will not be absorbed and assimilated into the bloodstream, displaying a condition called mal-absorption.

Just as the ballerina knows her cue when to step onto the stage, so do your digestive enzymes know when and how to interface with any given food. Yet, when the pH is out of balance, the enzymes retreat, as if waiting for their cue to tell them to "step onto the stage," to start participating in the digestive process. Our digestion requires appropriate timing, adjusted by the pH for the enzymes' activation and maximum effectiveness.

Most good nutritional diet books that address pH levels advocate eating more alkaline foods in order to avoid cellular acidity. Life in general doesn't respond very well when compartmentalized. Yet it instantly recognizes the fluidity of interrelated polarities, like yin and yang, without giving more weight and importance to either, by flowing within its totality. Acidity in itself isn't always a bad sign, and it certainly has its place within the body, particularly when it comes to our natural timing, the circadian rhythm. Rather than condemning one or the other extreme, I would like to educate you about how the interplay, with its exact timing, like the dancing ballerinas who finely tune their movements with the conductor's given cues, ultimately leads to a full experience of health.

A vital, organic, and alive nutrition is a huge part in the stabilization of the pH moderation. Unfortunately, the typical daily diet is geared for a fast lifestyle, which certainly adds to the internal physical confusion of our most intelligent system, the body, and only results in illness and concurrent symptomatologies.

A balanced pH of the blood is essential and critical for your life! As your body is and will always be your best friend, it will do anything to keep you alive. So, when the pH vacillates or is imbalanced, your body sacrifices the calcium in its bones to rescue it from its weakened state. This situation can set the stage for osteoporosis, often seen in women with diets full of acid food elements from red meat, soda, and excess sugar. Of course, antibiotics or steroids can have the same effect. Compensating for the lack of calcium with supplementation, while the daily nutritional intake is lacking most fundamental building blocks, isn't the answer here. When the pH is off, enzymes that are constructive can become destructive. Further, when the pH continues to be off kilter, oxygen delivery to the cells suffers and microbial-looking forms in the blood can change shape, mutate, or mirror pathogenicity and grow. You are the one who can change this! Before continuing with more information about the circadian rhythm, or inner body clock, here are some simple guidelines on how to balance your pH level easily and affordably.

Simple Kitchen Pharmacy to regulate your pH

If you are too acidic, you might add more cool showers to your daily regime. You may benefit greatly from a 6-oz. organic pineapple juice drink or other fresh fruit juice with no added artificial sugars (not cranberry juice) or any fresh vegetable juice. You can also add herb teas, like chamomile, peppermint, fenugreek, red clover, or hibiscus.

My favorite acid-reducer is a salt and baking soda bath, or Epson salt and baking soda bath. Take and dissolve 2 lb. salt and 2 lb. baking soda in a full bathtub. Take your time and soak at least for an hour!

The cheapest and easiest help comes in the form of pure, organic squeezed lemon juice mixed in water, best to be consumed on awakening and before your breakfast.

If you are too alkaline, take lots of hot baths and showers. A bath filled with 1 oz. dry mustard (do not stay in longer than 10 to 14 minutes) will wake you up in no time. You can also soak in a vinegar bath with 2 cups of vinegar to a full bathtub.

Drink unsweetened cranberry juice, best diluted in water. Herbal teas, like spearmint, shave grass, horsetail, raspberry leaf, and buchu can also be very beneficial. Eat a lot of sauerkraut, sour pickles, or olives, as well as low-stress proteins, like overnight soaked nuts and seeds. And take your dog out for a daily walk!

Although we may have heard about the pH level, and even know about its meaning of being too acidic or too alkaline, I am often asked which foods can be categorized as acid or alkaline. Here is a brief summary of available food choices:

Acid Food and Drink

LOWEST ACID FOODS

Processed honey, plums, processed fruits, juices, cooked spinach, kidney beans, string beans, pumpkin seeds, sunflower seeds, corn oil, sprouted wheat bread, brown rice, spelt, venison, eggs, butter, yoghurt, buttermilk, cottage cheese, and tea.

ACID FOODS

White sugar, brown sugar, sour cherries, rhubarb, potatoes (without skins), pinto beans, navy beans, lima beans, dried beans (mung, adzuki, pinto, kidney, garbanzo), white rice, corn, buckwheat, oats, rye, barley, bran, turkey, chicken, lamb, raw milk, milk (homogenized), coffee, bananas (green), blueberries, cereals (unrefined), cheeses, crackers (unrefined rye, rice, and wheat), cranberries, coconut (dry), egg (whites), eggs whole (cooked, hard), goat's milk (homogenized), honey (pasteurized), ketchup, and maple syrup (unprocessed).

MOST ACID FOODS

NutraSweet, Equal, Aspartame, Sweet'N Low (or any artificial sweetener), blackberries, cranberries, prunes, chocolate, peanuts, walnuts, wheat, white flour, breads, pastries, pasta, beef, pork, lamb, shellfish, cheese, homogenized milk, ice cream, beer, soft drinks, brown sugar, cereals (refined), chocolate, cigarettes and tobacco, coffee, cream of wheat (unrefined), custard (with white sugar), venison, drugs, fruit juices with sugar, and jams and jellies.

Alkaline Food and Drink

LOWEST ALKALINE FOODS

Raw honey, raw sugar, oranges, bananas, cherries, pineapple, peaches, avocados, carrots, tomatoes, fresh corn, mushrooms, cabbage, peas, potato skins, olives, tofu, chestnuts, canola oil, amaranth, millet, wild rice, quinoa, almonds, artichoke, Brussels sprouts, coconut (fresh), cucumber, eggplant, onions, pickles (homemade), radishes, sea salt, and spices.

ALKALINE FOODS

Maple syrup, rice syrup, dates, figs (fresh), melons, raisins, grapes, kiwi, blueberries, apples, pears (less sweet), okra, squash, green beans, beets, celery, lettuce, zucchini, sweet potato, carob, almonds, flax seed oil, alfalfa sprouts, apricots, avocados, bananas (ripe), currants, garlic,

Core Body

grapefruit, grapes (less sweet), guavas, herbs (leafy green), nectarine, peaches (sweet), peas (fresh, sweet), pumpkin (sweet), and sea salt.

MOST ALKALINE FOODS

Stevia, lemons, limes, watermelon, cantaloupe, grapefruit, mango, papaya, asparagus, onions, garlic, parsley, raw spinach, broccoli, vegetable juices, olive oil, celery, kelp, seaweed, seedless grapes (sweet), and watercress.

OPTIMAL TIME TO EAT

The body thrives the most when given the appropriate nutrients at the optimal time. This built-in body clock facilitates the metabolism of your food, the storage of the nutrients, the release of its energy, or the detoxification of its by-products with its final elimination. It is therefore important to know when to eat proteins and when to consume carbohydrates.

Envision a graph with a wave line going up and down that indicates the time phases within a 24-hour cycle. During the second part of the night our body resides in an alkaline state. At about 4:00 a.m. we enter an acid state, which peaks at about 9:00 a.m. and declines in the early afternoon hours. At around 3:30 to 4:00 p.m. we thrive on the peak alkaline swing, which again changes around midnight into its acid swing only to return to an alkaline state through the latter part of the night. This cycle will complete itself in our return to an acid state in the early hours of the morning. Due to this rhythmic interchange of acidity and alkalinity within the body, it is essential to feed our cells with the appropriately timed cellular pH food.

Our protein enzyme reservoir works best early in the day, as it was replenished and rested by the night before. The large intestines start to go to work around 5:00 to 7:00 a.m., followed by stomach activity from 7:00 to 9:00 a.m., when the most active digestive processes occur. On waking, the body moves into the acid state, indicating the body is ready to move and meet the day. With all the digestive processes and enzymes in place, it is a perfect time to introduce proteins. Proteins are generally much more difficult to process than carbohydrates and require a strong and effective digestive system, which is much better equipped in the morning.

Protein foods, like meat, fish, eggs, or organic sprouted tofu with fresh or slightly steamed vegetables and green salads are best introduced to the body early in the day, benefitting us all during our active and productive phases. Carbohydrates and alkaline foods are best eaten with the evening meal, as they are more sedative in their effect.

If you eat your breakfast before 9:00 a.m., just before the peak of the acid phase, your digestion process will still slightly pull to the alkaline side, which also stabilizes your blood sugar level. The initial digestion of the vegetables in the meal also causes a slight alkaline pull on the system within 30 minutes of eating. Hours later, the ingested proteins from breakfast will create a mild acid terrain in the body and support the entire metabolism during its alkaline swing in the later afternoon. The common breakfast, consisting of fruits, cereals, sugar, milk, and toast topped with the cup of coffee and consumed by most adults and children as they rush to work or school, swing us back into an alkaline state too soon, resulting in tiredness and the feeling that we've run out of steam by early afternoon. This partly happens due to the quick digestion of fruits and rendering of alkalizing minerals, which block the active and productive morning acid phase within the body. So often, by 3:00 or 4:00 p.m. (when the liver becomes active) we then find ourselves craving sweets or reaching for the next cup of coffee, just to keep us going for another two to three hours at work.

In *The Pro-Vita! Plan for Optimal Nutrition* Dr. Tips explains: "Eating protein properly for breakfast works to stabilize the natural pH swing. Eight hours later, in the mid afternoon, the proteins have been digested, assimilated and are being used. At this time, the body pH is swinging into an alkaline pH. Then the proteins buffer that swing, preventing alkalosis and low blood sugar, thus preventing fatigue or the need for sweets and coffee."

Talking about when to eat proteins and carbohydrates often incites comments like: "I can't imagine eating a plate of eggs or salmon with vegetables for breakfast! What about my muesli or my cereal?" If you cannot eat a substantial meal at 6:00 a.m., please feel free to enjoy your smoothie with your favorite berries and fruits first, but start eating a protein meal with a variety of vegetables by around 9:00 to 10:00 am, as well as for lunch. And who says that your protein meal has to be all meat or fish? There are plenty of proteins in vegetables, too. As I am a vegetarian from birth I have learned to extract more proteins out of my vegetables to replenish my overall protein pool (with the help of supplements). You do not necessarily have to eat animal proteins if you don't wish to do so. This opinion is not generally accepted, however, even among nutritionists, and is solely based on my personal experience as a life-long vegetarian.

To balance your pH levels naturally with nutrition alone, it is vital to understand these guidelines. You now understand that on waking you enter into a natural acidic state, leaving the alkaline state from the previous night. If you eat a breakfast comprised of fruits, sugar, and grains, this approach causes an excess of alkalinity in the body too much and too soon. In order to avoid this out-of-proportion swing, you can now stabilize your natural acid state with a wonderful pH-balanced diet nurturing you and building your cells throughout the early part of the day. This is harmonious balance in action!

In the afternoon, eight hours later, the digested proteins, now converted into amino acids, are available for metabolic activity to stabilize the alkaline swing that peaks around 3:00 to 4:00 p.m.

In the evening, being in an alkaline state, you then want to offer your body more acidic food like carbohydrates to harmonize your alkaline terrain. This is the time you can enjoy your pasta dish with vegetables and a salad, for example.

As the body doesn't provide the essential enzymes for protein digestion in the evening, it is best not to eat any protein, like meat or nuts, at your evening meal. The proteins, the steak or the handful of almonds, will not be properly digested or completely metabolized during sleep and end up piling up as toxins in your blood and lymph. Have you ever wondered why you toss and turn around in your bed unable to fall asleep after a Thanksgiving dinner? It all has to do with a congested lymphatic system that really wanted to go to sleep, too. Unfortunately, most of our protein meals are consumed in the evening, when the family comes together after a long day of work and school. So, remember, proteins eaten late in the day become toxic in the body.

> The primary rule for every diet plan should be:
> DO NOT MIX MAJOR PORTIONS OF PROTEINS
> WITH CARBOHYDRATES/STARCH AT THE SAME MEAL

Try to eat your proteins early in the day in combination with fresh or lightly steamed vegetables or a variety of fresh salads. The body requires these vegetables, as they provide the needed food enzymes that help break down the given proteins. Enzymes are made out of amino acids, the building blocks of proteins. If we are low in our protein reservoirs, our ability to digest and assimilate proteins is severely hindered. During the day, avoid all carbohydrates, particularly the mixing of proteins and carbohydrates. This means your turkey sandwich at lunch would be not the best idea. As the body intelligently fights for its survival, it chooses the sugar or carbohydrates first, and leaves the proteins undigested. It is best to stop eating all proteins after 2:00 to 3:00 p.m. After that, consume all carbohydrates with a variety of vegetables or fresh salads in the evening, leaving out any protein. Carbohydrates actually calm the brain through the release of endorphins.

Did you know that eating proteins in combination with carbohydrates is the major cause of cholesterol problems? I have seen patients normalize their cholesterol readings solely by changing their dietary habits and without the aid of medication. Did you know that the condition of having undigested proteins, called protein toxicity, is a direct cause of cancer today? Again, your health is determined by what you eat and at what time you enjoy your meals. In the words of Lao Tzu's: "Nature does not hurry, yet everything is accomplished."

Core Body

As soon as you start paying attention to these basic and simple guidelines, your body will not only function at its optimal level, but you will become distinctly in tune with the natural rhythm of your body. You will learn how and when to dance with your body. It's a beautiful dance!

> Life is not about waiting for the storm to pass,
> It's about learning how to dance in the rain.
> —Unknown

Lack of Energy and Cellular Inflammation Breaks the Dance

> Everything is energy and that's all there is to it. Match the frequency
> of the reality you want and you cannot help but get that reality.
> It can be no other way. This is not philosophy. This is physics.
>
> —Albert Einstein

Your journey of transformative healing now takes you deep into the interior of your body. Choose a safe and familiar place for your next dance. This can be your living room or a favorite place in Nature, anywhere you feel alive and grounded. The music begins with a soft and gentle rhythm. You take a scarf or a blindfold and place it over your eyes, allowing you to see only yourself and your body with your "inner eyes." In this way you can turn your focus inward, rather than be distracted by external images. As you relax and fall into your body, your arms and torso gently start to sway, following the harmonic tunes of the song.

Allowing yourself to feel your body in this way might be quite a new experience and it might take some time to become familiar with this different relationship with yourself and your body.

As your vision turns inward, you suddenly see and feel your inner world with all its organs, tissues, and fluids. Your liver might feel sluggish or your digestive system congested, whereas your heart might feel joyful and light. Now go a step further. Try to see and feel your cells. What do they look like? Are they happy or are they struggling? Choose an organ, perhaps your heart, and tune into its cells. Are they clogged, congested, asking for your help? Or do you sense your heart-felt cells radiating compassion and love? Do your cells have a color, like flaming red, meaning they might be inflamed, or are they a cooling blue, meaning they are calm and functioning well?

You are still dancing, and as you deeply connect with your interior world your dance slowly takes on the external form of this internal dialogue. Your movements radiate the frequency of the inner state of your body, whether in health or illness. Your dance now becomes a conversation with your body. Make it a creative and joyful conversation, a conversation you will always remember! No one is watching, so dance!

As you delve deeper into your most interior terrain and get closer to your core Self, the mind starts letting go of its control strategies. At this point, it simply cannot stop the unfolding process as you close the gap between your heart and feelings. You literally drop out of the intellectual and analytical parts of your mind and fall into your heart, your true brain of awareness and consciousness.

Whenever I explain the basic principles of cellular biology, a visible struggle between the mind and body appears immediately on the patient's face. It is not the lack of intellectual understanding that seems to fuel this scenario, but a deep-seated fear of the unknown. In entering the interior vastness of yourself, you will be faced with who you are and how your body functions day after day. In this way, you bridge the chasm of yourself and your physical body as it merges into a unified container called "You." This book presents the most cutting-edge scientific research in simple terms and in easy and accessible language to help you clear the way of any unfounded fears and reservations in exploring this unknown territory: your body.

It all starts with energy! Humans, animals, plants, and everything else connected to this planet Earth are all vibrational beings infused with energy. Everything in the universe is in a constant state of vibration. Solid, liquid, or gas, everything is made of energy, and all forms of energy are constantly moving and vibrating at a subatomic level. Even intangible substances like sounds, color, and thoughts, and emotions resonate with individual frequencies. Certain thoughts carry certain frequencies that will resonate with other humans who have similar thoughts, or with animals or plants that express the same frequency of thought patterns. Conversely, disharmony occurs when different resonating vibrations clash. The song and the dance are now out of tune and out of rhythm.

We are energy and energy is everything! This primal life energy is called ch'i in Chinese Traditional Medicine, and prana in Ayurveda, a traditional medicine native to India. It is responsible for all our life processes, mental, emotional, and spiritual. Energy causes what happens around us. During the day, the sun gives out light energy and heat energy. At night, street lamps use electrical energy to light our way. When a car drives by, it is powered by gasoline (or perhaps electricity), a type of stored energy. The food we eat is energy we use to work and play. Yet, perhaps with the exception of energy in the form of light, energy is not a thing, per se; rather, energy refers to a condition or state of a thing.

We often speak of energy as something that can be stored, bought, sold, and transported. But the condition of "having energy" is never created anew, and never destroyed, only passed from one object to another. In this way, energy is unique among conditions. Energy is always in movement. It flows with the ability to change its shape and experience and is never stagnant. In terms of physics, every living and nonliving object is composed of tiny particles of matter. These particles are in constant motion. This motion and dance creates your energy! Energy exists in all matter and its main source is the universe itself.

In Traditional Chinese Medicine, a sick person is described as having a "congested energy," and a healthy person is described as having a "circulating flowing energy." When your cosmic, mental, emotional, and physical energy fields are negatively affected, you feel the impact in the form of symptoms like pain, fever, and heat—the initial signs of a congested physical situation. The body, a true miracle, is self-programmed, self-directing, self-governing, self-repairing, and self-healing. Furthermore, it is able to cleanse itself, defend itself, and is certainly highly self-sufficient. Therefore, with the proper energy supply through healthy nutrition and available cellular energy, your body, from its denser to its most minutely refined parts, can shine once again.

Dr. Jack Tips reminds us that, "Energy is the foundation of health. Energy and health are so deeply allied in an interchangeable cause-and-effect relationship, that one can say, energy is synonymous with health. If your body can make energy, it is healthy. If your body is healthy (properly nourished), it can make plenty of energy."

Your body needs cellular energy to live, breathe, act, feel, think, and digest your food. Cellular energy provides the muscle power to walk, the ability to sleep, and to support all the body's incredible daily functions. Without cellular energy, nothing works! In today's world, filled with an onslaught of external toxicity from air, water, and soil pollution, radiation, chemicals, pesticides, drugs, and a generally non-nutritional diet, our cells do not get what they need in order to implement their individual tasks. The result of this massive global change manifests within our bodies as an alarming lack of cellular energy, which is directly linked to the occurrence of most diseases. When the cells work at their optimal capacity, all our tissues, organs, and glands also work to their best and highest levels. When our cells feel energized and alive, they communicate with all the other cells in the body, creating an incredible network system of youthful vitality and adaptability. But this social network and interrelationship within our cells is profoundly interrupted when we are ill, as the cells just don't feel like talking anymore. Sound familiar? After a bad day at work when we feel tired and exhausted of energy, most of us want to be quiet for a while before we decide to engage in a lively conversation.

Our bodies have multiple ways to produce the energy we need to survive. Human beings derive energy from the sun through the photosynthesis of plants. The plants turn light into energy and produce the prime nutritional molecules of sugar, fats, and proteins. Consuming plant matter nurtures and energizes our bodies with this life-giving, converted sun-energy. This is the reason you must include an abundant variety of fresh, organic fruits, and vegetables into your daily diet.

Core Body

So, where in the body is all this energy created? Inside your cells are specific power-generating organelles called mitochondria. These powerhouses are necessary for the life of each cell within the body (except red blood cells), and each cell can contain over 2,500 mitochondria in its single nucleus that work tirelessly to keep us alive and healthy. A lack of cellular energy is synonymous with cellular aging, which means aging prematurely or becoming ill. Without an efficient cellular energy production, the body has a tendency to retain toxins, because it simply does not have the energy to burn them up, chemically alter them, or otherwise support the detoxification process. Energy keeps us alive, lets us function throughout our lives, protects us from external stimuli, repairs and protects the cell's DNA, detoxifies metabolic wastes, enables the cells to communicate with each other, supports our metabolic, hormonal, and nerve transmission processes, and, most of all, stimulates our immune system in meeting today's health challenges.

When there is a lack of cellular energy inevitable problems arise. Not only does the body age more rapidly, but tissues degenerate, hormones become less effective, arteries harden, cellular communication becomes garbled, inflammation becomes chronic, fat gets stored, the brain becomes sluggish, the immune system gets confused, and pathogens start to create their own world inside the body. If you do not have enough fuel for your body, the mitochondria shut down, go dormant; they simply do not want to go to work anymore. With a nutritious, healthy, and vital diet, the mitochondria are normally able to create the needed fuel. Yet even with the most optimal nutrition available today, these powerhouses do not receive what they need in order to create the life-energy due to the onslaught of external and internal toxicity with which we are faced. As the body ages, the number of functional mitochondria decreases, indicating it is running out of steam. That is why elderly people are the most affected and experience less physical energy and vitality. The decline of these mitochondria might not be blamed on time and age, but on the lack of vital energy, which is needed to protect, repair, and maintain these cellular processes. You need energy to dance and your cells need energy to make you dance!

Core Body

In biochemical terms, the energy produced by the mitochondria is called Adenosine TriPhosphate, or ATP. ATP is the body's chemical energy of life. The same principle is at work in plants, which store the energy harvested via the light reaction by forming the same ATP chemical, the compound used by cells for energy storage. This chemical is made of the nucleotide adenine, bonded to a ribose sugar and to three phosphate groups. This molecule is very similar to the building blocks of our DNA.

Today, our larger world economic, social, and health-related crises right through the crises we are experiencing on a physical cellular level are based on one common denominator, the deficiency and lack of free and clean energy in its crude and unrefined form. Unless we provide planet Earth and our bodies a proper and balanced nutrition and the collaborating cellular energy, we will continue to live on a principle based on borrowed time and false expectations.

This current gloomy global situation is an eye-opening mirror image of our poor and divided relationship toward our bodies and life in general. In the same way the world lives on borrowed wealth, printing new dollar bills on demand by starving out third world countries, so are we as individuals abusing and using up our cellular energy every day that we live. If you do not add money to your bank account, it will not refill itself automatically. Eventually, if your spending exceeds your deposits you will reach a zero balance. But at least if worse comes to worst financially you can declare bankruptcy, and can start your life over again from scratch. It may not be fun, but it's doable. Your physical energy, however, does not work like a bank. This energy "account" arrives only once—not twice—and comes in one single parcel. Your energy reservoirs need replenishing every day, day after day, with life-giving nutrition and conscious mindfulness, if it is to stay vital and strong.

We live in one of the most exciting times in history. Not only is much of the latest scientific research walking a path alongside spiritual consciousness, but also humankind is recognizing the value of holistic vibrational medicine and its respected place in the greater medical context. Switzerland, for example, advocated for and has declared homeopathy a beneficial and effective medicine to be fully acknowledged by its politicians and parliament.

We as a human species, along with the animal and plant kingdoms, can only sustain ourselves if we start exploring the fundamental principle of energy production in our bodies and the planet. If we continue to rape the planet of its resources without giving back in the same way we are raping our bodies of their life-giving energy, expecting them to work day-in and day-out without stopping to contemplate how to refuel these magnificent creations, our struggles will only increase. Our future healing must culminate in a harmonious convergence where the needs of the planet and of humankind meet via a harmonious interchange that does not deplete the other's energy reserves. Humanity must shift from living on Earth to living with Her, and mirror this shift within by living alongside the body to living with the body.

More and more scientific research is being published regarding the core links between global and universal energy patterns. Evidence of this interconnectedness can be seen in films like *Thrive: What On Earth Will It Take?*, a feature-length documentary at www.thrivemovement.com. All over the world we, the stewards of this planet, are exploring the search for the creation of free and renewable energy. Yet the same energy crisis in our economic and Earth changes is powerfully reflected in our bodies' physical cells, starving and depleted of their prime energy supply. It is time to herald a new era in the relationship between your body and the life-giving cellular energy it craves.

Let's return to our depleted mitochondria for a moment. Once damaged, the mitochondria experience something similar to a nuclear reactor meltdown. This meltdown causes long-term damage in the body, including cellular malfunction, destruction, and aberrant cellular behavior. Deficient of energy, and in the midst of a changed cellular environment, the cells begin to behave differently. Sometimes they become confused and lose sight of their goals. Sometimes they go rogue. The ones that do are the most invasive invaders and destroyers of mitochondria, electrons called free radicals. With a short supply in oxygen and fuel, the mitochondrias' own free radicals, the body's by-products in the making of energy, damage independent genetic material. Since the mitochondria carry their own genetic codes, they require energy to repair and maintain them. With an ongoing onslaught of environmental pollutants and metabolic toxins, this necessary oxygen supply is interrupted and our cells are left tired ... exhausted ... burnt out.

The principle of how environmental change affects our cellular behavior applies here more than ever. This is a very important point, as you, with your capacity for freedom of choice, can change your environment and thereby influence the well-being of your entire biochemical structure. As soon as your body receives its necessary energy supply, your cells can begin to repair their DNA via enzymes and glycopeptides, similar to glycoprotein, but built of smaller proteins (amino acid chains) and thus more accessible to the cells.

Practically every cell in our bodies has miniature power plants called mitochondria where glucose and other simple sugars mix with oxygen and burn to keep us warm, active and alive. If the fuel mix is correct, it contains a mixture of mostly glucose/ribose, a tiny amount of amino acids and fat, and the right amount of oxygen for power combustion. When this mixture is present, then the cellular life-fires burn properly, providing stable health and optimal energy. Everything is fine as long as these elements can be maintained. —Dr. Jack Tips

As discussed, as the mitochondria create energy, or ATP, they also create free radical electrons, a harmful by-product of the process. To counteract this course, the mitochondria also produce antioxidants, which immediately set about capturing and neutralizing the free radicals. Your body always works in unison with the rest of you; as your best friend, it always has a back-up plan to keep you alive, particularly during a crisis, such as when an organ starts to fail. Unless the mitochondria receive an adequate energy supply, however, they will not be able to control this free radical outbreak sufficiently to offset their own demise at the hand of their own metabolic by-products.

Today, we all suffer from an alarmingly increasing amount of free radical damage, the first step in manifesting disease. I therefore encourage you to change your nutritional diet to a life-nurturing, energy-producing experience that will keep you alive, vibrant, and young. Biochemically speaking, the mitochondria might be compared to the body's fountain of youth, rejuvenating the cellular world with boundless and vital energy. As long as we bombard our bodies with xenobiotic toxins from pesticides to domestic chemicals, heavy metals, vaccinations, food additives, cell phones, radiation from airport body scanners and x-rays, nuclear radiation, smoke detectors, and radon gas (to name only some of the offenders) we not only continue to choke ourselves off from a clean oxygen supply, but choke off our cells from the energy supply critical to their survival.

But this decline and malfunction of the mitochondria has an even more devastating effect in that it also affects our DNA, and consequently the very identity of our cells. If the situation has reached this point, the cells have long forgotten their names and functions and no longer know where they belong.

Our symptoms, diseases, and ailing bodies are primarily expressions of a fundamental lack of cellular energy. It's as simple as that. Although conceptually basic, and even obvious to some of us, it has taken the medical establishment many decades to even consider this linkage in relationship to our declining health. The body responds immediately to the production of energy and the proper amount of energy to influence and stimulate all the organs and tissues, including the brain. Given what it needs, the brain will function at its optimal level and provide you with a clear mind and sharp memory and your digestion will receive and assimilate your food rhythmically and successfully. Your nerves will transport accumulated information via the most selective and smooth transmission. Your overall metabolism will function at its best; your hormones will finally communicate and work with each other in a balanced manner; your muscles will contract and expand perfectly during exercise; and your sexual desire will be balanced and well received. Not to mention that your immune system will know when and how to join the party, and your detoxification system that will make sure that toxins and metabolic accumulated waste products are chemically altered and eliminated on a continuous basis.

Core Body

When the mitochondria do not produce enough energy, their capacity to release waste products is diminished and the cell's capacity to receive nutrients is hampered. This means that nothing goes in or out of the cell membranes. If cellular energy production falls below those required to sustain life, you die. This is the moment your dance comes to its end! So, as you can see, the creation of life-giving energy in the form of ATP is paramount to optimal health, planetary sustainability, and life itself.

A truly healthy person radiates an aura of wellness and light. We might compliment her by saying, "You look so radiant and healthy!" Have you ever wondered what it is about this person that causes you feel—or actually see—this radiance? We all have seen the beautiful view of the sun over the ocean as it sets over the horizon as the day draws to its close. Often, just before the sun finally hits the horizon, we might see white, sparkly phosphoric lights flickering and dancing on the water's surface. This is called phosphoric light—and you are made of just such sweet and joyful light particles, which are actually ATP molecules that split into combustible energy units of Adenosine DiPhosphate (ADP) and phosphorus when the body requests the release of some of its stored energy. When ATP "explodes" into ADP, the result is tiny explosions of phosphorescent light.

Millions and millions of such tiny lights blink on in the body in the form of the energy that keeps us alive and inspires us to accomplish all our daily functions. The body's inherent intelligence decides where the requested energy supply will be transported. The heart might use the energy for its muscular contractions, the leg for the muscles to contract and expand, the kidneys to filter the blood or make Vitamin D, the brain for thought processes, the intestines for absorption, or the immune system for invading stimulants. You are a being created into your individual form by energy, and only energy in all its multifaceted expressions keeps you alive and well.

It can never be stated enough that none of our bodies are exempt from the environmental toxicity and global changes with which we are bombarded today. The thousands of toxins, vaccinations filled with carcinogenic components, food additives, drugs, and generally poisonous lifestyles are severely depleting cellular energy production on a global scale. Just think about the recent nuclear reactor meltdown in Fukushima, Japan, now polluting the entire globe with radioactive elements such as Strontium-90, Cesium-137, Iodine-131 and Plutonium-239, or the Deepwater Horizon oil spill off the Gulf of Mexico now polluting our oceans. Sadly, these global catastrophes mirror all too precisely the situation occurring in our bodies, particularly in regard to the damage and death of our cells.

For a brief moment, step away from your body and try to see a wider perspective or the bigger picture. Major global environmental changes profoundly affecting the Arctic and Antarctic are transforming enormous masses of ice, frozen for thousands of years, into water. We cannot even comprehend what such a shift will do to the planet over the long run, although I think we can all agree it will be significant and we will all be affected. What we do know is that if current trends thinning the Arctic ice ocean to half its size since 1980 continue, we will see nothing but open ocean by the year 2020. The days of continuous sheets of ice and frolicking polar bears could soon be a thing of the past.

For animals and people in that changing terrain we hope that life will go on, at least for those who are able to adapt and thrive. But the loss of sea ice is not something happening "out there." Whatever is happening in the Arctic is happening to the whole planet to one degree or another, and to our bodies—all the way down to the smallest cell of our biology. As the environment changes, so does the behavior of our cells. A toxic environment creates toxic behavior. To cleanse, nurture, invigorate, and rebuild the body, we must use the most effective and natural treatments, remedies, and supplements to pave the way to an easier adaptation and transition. Remember, the ability to adapt to environmental changes is the determining factor of all health.

The scientific and medical community acknowledges that there are some diseases that are primarily caused by an initial lack of cellular energy, rather than individual symptomatologies. The list of so-called "mitochondria diseases" includes, but is not limited to, Alzheimer's, dementia, arteriosclerosis, ataxia, atherosclerosis, autism, blindness, congestive heart disease, cancer with metastasis, liver cirrhosis, Crohn's disease, deafness, type 2 diabetes, epilepsy, fatigue, fibromyalgia, hypercholesterolemia, hypertension, neurogastrointestinal encephalopathy, insulin resistance and general hormone resistance (estrogen, progesterone, testosterone, leptin, thyroxin), irritable bowel syndrome, kidney failure, systemic lupus, multiple sclerosis, muscular dystrophy, myasthenia gravis, obesity, Parkinson's, retinitis pigmentosa, rheumatoid arthritis, strokes, and Wilson's thyroid syndrome.

We know that most cellular damage is caused by free radicals with resultant cellular inflammation. Going back in time to your high-school chemistry class, you may remember that the most important structural feature of an atom that determines its chemical behavior is the number of electrons in its outer shell. Atoms often complete their outer shells by sharing electrons with other atoms. By sharing these electrons, the atoms are bound together, creating a safe and stable environment for the molecule. Normally these bonds don't split in a way that leaves a molecule with an odd and unpaired electron. But when weak bonds split, free radicals are formed. Free radicals, which are very unstable and react quickly with other compounds, attempt to capture the needed electron to gain stability. You might say that free radicals display a mean nature as they attack the nearest stable molecule, literally stealing its own needed electron. With the loss of its electron, the molecule mutates into a free radical itself, thus beginning a chain reaction. The process, once begun, can cause a domino effect and ultimately destroy the living cell.

Some free radicals are naturally created by the body's own metabolism. Sometimes the immune system purposefully creates them to neutralize viruses and bacteria. However, environmental changes and toxicity profoundly affect their presence. A healthy body can handle these bad guys, but if antioxidants are unavailable, or if the free-radical production becomes excessive, damage often occurs. With age and less cellular energy production, free radical damage accumulates throughout the body. For this reason, we really don't want to provide a physical terrain that attracts and benefits these destructive elements.

The best and most efficient way to quench free radicals is the consumption of antioxidants like vitamins C and E. Antioxidants neutralize free radicals by donating one of their own electrons, therefore ending their kidnapping spree. Because the antioxidant nutrients are already stable in either form, they can resist pressure to become free radicals by donating and electron to the cause. In fact, they act as wonderful scavengers, preventing cell and tissue damage that can lead to disease. If you add 5 to 8 servings of fruits and vegetables and natural supplementation to your daily balanced diet, you are sure to set the stage for your body to heal, particularly regarding inflammatory diseases, and promote longevity.

Understanding Cellular Inflammation

We all understand what it means to experience an inflamed shoulder or suffer from an inflamed knee joint. Yet there are two types of inflammation. The first is called classical inflammation, which generates the inflammatory response associated with heat, redness, swelling, pain, and degenerative tissue changes. For example, perhaps you cut your foot stepping on a piece of glass on your recent camping trip. If it turned into a nasty infection it would have been due to damage to the tissue and cells from accumulating bacteria. As the body is always ready to help, its mast cells released histamine and cytokines (cell-signaling protein molecules that increase during trauma or infection), alarming the entire body of this emergency. At the site of the wound, capillaries released immune cells, stimulating the body to get ready for the necessary defensive move. Then, wonderful macrophages (white blood cells that eat foreign material) attacked the bacteria. Other friends also arrived at the scene, called neutrophils, whose job it was to engulf the bacteria and damaged cells. Yet another group of helpers, white blood cells, secrete interleukins, set the stage for the body to experience a fever, while releasing certain chemicals to support the whole process. Once the emergency was completely over, platelets (cells that circulate in the blood and clot to keep us from bleeding), fibrin (a fibrous, non-globular protein involved in the clotting of blood), and other many other helpful agents contributed to your overall wound healing, making sure you were on your feet again in no time.

The other type of inflammation is called cellular inflammation, which expresses itself below the perception of pain. We are not aware of, nor do we feel, cellular inflammation, yet it is the most destructive situation we face relative to disease. Cellular inflammation is the initiating cause of most chronic diseases. An unbelievable 80% of all doctor visits are for issues related to chronic diseases! Initially, inflammation occurs when the body attempts to defend itself against harmful pathogens, like a chronic, persistent bacteria or virus. This situation may be initiated by an army of free radicals that were launched when as we consumed a daily diet of foods made with processed vegetable oils, like French fries and chips, powdered milk, powdered coffee creamer, high-fat salad dressings, and the whole spectrum of processed foods. The stimulus might be an allergy to wheat and gluten that inflames the intestines, or a low-grade, lingering infection. It might also be created by an accumulation of floating heavy metals and pesticides/chemicals in the body. If you have ever experienced an injury that was followed by a low-grade ongoing infection like an unresolved root canal procedure, systemic cellular inflammation may be the result. Remember, your teeth are directly connected and interlinked with the meridians, the energy channels of your entire system.

This ongoing, or chronic, state of inflammation also occurs when the body's natural healing process goes too far and results in the destruction of healthy parts of the body like joints and blood vessels. Then we speak of an autoimmune, or self-attacking, situation. Once the immune system goes into overdrive, it literally believes that the causes of infection or cellular toxicity will never be fully removed. When this happens, the process of cellular inflammation doesn't quit, and white blood cells continue to enter the tissue even though there is no need for them anymore.

If you do not feel the actual smoldering pain, it may not occur to you that you are ill, but the internal fire quietly burning inside of you is upsetting the delicate balance among all your major bodily systems, from the endocrine system to the central nervous system, the digestive to the cardiovascular and respiratory systems. In a healthy body these systems communicate with each other clearly. But that essential communication becomes distorted when chronic inflammation is at the root of the problem. Today, even the orthodox medical community recognizes the connection between hypertension and the increased risk of Alzheimer's disease and between sufferers of rheumatoid arthritis and high rates of sudden cardiac death. It is clear that such ailments are all connected on a fundamental level: the level of cellular inflammation.

❦

In February, 2004 *Time Magazine* educated us about inflammation, calling it "The Secret Killer." This article clearly stated that the subject of inflammation has become one of the hottest areas of medical research today. For example, cellular inflammation destabilizes cholesterol deposits in the coronary arteries and is the true leading cause of heart attacks and, potentially, strokes.

Chronic inflammation has a damaging effect on arteries, which can lead to high cholesterol, heart attacks, and strokes. Microorganisms cause inflammation within the blood vessels by creating a lesion that attacks the inside of the arteries. Although immune cells are dispatched to fight the inflammation and cholesterol is laid down over the wound like a Band-Aid, under the Band-Aid the inflammation is still active. In time, the Band-Aid bulges and a small part of the blood vessel gives way. OMG! The wound, now enlarged, needs to be plugged—and fast! What it needs is a blood clot, like a cork for a wine bottle. But what happens when the blood clot breaks loose and travels to the brain? If the clot gets big enough, a stroke is the only likely eventuality. If the clot goes to the heart, a heart attack is the result.

Orthodox medicine still believes that statin, the best-selling drug worldwide that reduces high cholesterol, is the answer to this problem. But understanding our Band-Aid example, you now can see why suppressing cholesterol production is not a good way to address this problem. Statins may have anti-inflammatory properties, yet their side effects override their beneficial properties in the long run. Statins come with a price to pay! Not only does their use bypass the true cause of high cholesterol and arterial plaque, but also side effects, which include muscle weakness and mental problems. Statins do not quench the interior smoldering fire, nor do they bring about a true and long-lasting cure. In fact, as early as 2008, the Mayo Clinic Proceedings stated that researchers had found that fish oils and red yeast rice supplements lowered bad cholesterol better than statins!

Did you know that half of all heart attacks occur in people with normal cholesterol levels? As imaging techniques have improved, we now know that most of the dangerous plaque wasn't nearly enough to cause many initial heart attacks. When scientists researched this phenomenon, they soon realized that it was cellular inflammation causing those deposits to burst and trigger the clots massive enough to cut off the coronary blood supply.

Dr. Paul Ridker, cardiologist at Brigham and Women's Hospital in Boston, Massachusetts, has done ground-breaking work in this arena, proving that inflammatory reaction is the responsible factor in bursting plaque. By 1997, Dr. Ridker and his colleagues had shown that healthy middle-aged men with the highest CRP levels (C-reactive protein, indicating inflammation via a blood test), were three times as likely to suffer a heart attack in the next six years as were those with the lowest CRP levels. If you experience atherosclerosis or the possibility for arterial plaque, do not blame your high cholesterol or your general cardiovascular situation. Instead, start your core healing by tackling your chronic cellular inflammation.

Dr. Dwight Lundell is a heart surgeon who conducted over 5,000 open-heart surgeries. Dr. Lundell reports: "Despite the fact that 25% of the population takes extensive statin medications, and despite the fact we have reduced the fat content of our diets, more Americans will die this year of heart disease than ever before. Simply stated, without inflammation being present in the body, there is no way that cholesterol would accumulate in the wall of the blood vessel and cause heart disease and strokes. Without inflammation, cholesterol would move freely throughout the body as nature intended it. It is inflammation that causes cholesterol to become trapped."

Dr. Lundell also refers to the fact that cellular inflammation is caused by the consumption of prepared and processed foods that trip the inflammation switch more and more, little by little, each day. Our human body is not designed to, nor can it, process foods with large amounts of sugar and soaked in omega-6 oils. The typically imbalanced ratio of omega-3, -6, and -9 to omega-6 oils consumed today contributes to the inflammatory process of the cell membrane, which produces the cytokines that directly cause inflammation. It all goes back to your plate!

Cellular inflammation affects your entire body as it chews up nerve cells, as evidenced in the brains of Alzheimer's patients. It may even foster the proliferation of abnormal cells and facilitate their transmission onto cancer.

In 1860, renowned pathologist Rudolf Virchov speculated that cancerous tumors arise at the site of chronic inflammation. Today, researchers are working diligently to explore the possibility that cellular mutation and inflammation are mutually reinforcing processes within the body, and are finding more and more evidence for the supposition that inflammation plays a much more significant role in chronic disease than they initially believed.

Cellular chronic inflammation becomes the engine that drives many of the most feared diseases of our population. It also has a major influence on type 2 diabetes. The complex interplay between insulin and fat, either in the diet or in the large folds under the skin, create inflammatory cytokines and prostaglandins (all chemicals that further inflammation), particularly with weight gain. Cellular inflammation may be present in the early stages of autoimmune diseases, like multiple sclerosis as well, where the destruction of tissue contributes to permanent nerve damage.

One of the most rapidly growing diseases is certainly asthma, which is clearly and solely an inflammatory condition. As the person experiences tightening in the chest, the muscles around the airways of the lungs squeeze together or tighten. The actual inflammation may not be experienced as such, yet the airways are chronically inflamed, swollen, and irritated. Inflammation can directly reduce the amount of air that we can take in and breathe out.

Core Body

Women may be curious to learn that our monthly hormonal issues, from mood swings to menstrual cramps, may have less to do with the production of the hormonal glands and more to do with polluted cell membranes' resisting the hormonal messengers. Polluted cell membranes can stimulate both hormone and insulin resistance and more. Symptoms of chronic inflammation often become more apparent during and after menopause, and hormonal changes leading up to menopause often contribute to the dreaded weight gain. When you gain weight, fat cells become more biochemically active as they continue to churn out inflammatory compounds. Extra fat cells, especially around the middle of the body (so-called "belly fat"), add to systemic inflammation by creating extra cytokines and C-reactive proteins (the indicators for cellular inflammation). One more reason to lose the extra pounds now!

Some of this extra weight comes from excess calories, no doubt, but some comes from toxins stored in the fat cells. Our bodies have become dumping grounds for the tens of thousands of toxic compounds that invade our everyday world, setting the stage for an overall slow decline in health.

The Environmental Protection Agency (EPA) estimates there are more than 20,000 chemicals we might put in our bodies that they cannot metabolize. Incapable of excretion from the body, these chemicals find their way into the liver, and then migrate to fat cells for storage. Studies show that most of us have between 400 to 800 chemical residues stored in our cells.

Again, this is why following a yearly physical maintenance program that includes a thorough detoxification protocol is so important. Detox serves as a prime rejuvenation tool and support for the body (to be discussed in the next chapter). Detrimental toxins need to be released; they have to be skillfully escorted out of the body, however, or they merely resettle again in other parts. An experienced heath care practitioner is invaluable here, as the various organs of the body need to be well supported throughout this vital process.

Core Body

As we go further, this deep-seated inflammation can affect the gums, nail beds, and the small intestines to the colon, as well as the space outside and inside of your cells, and influence the entire body. Cellular inflammation is a severe terrain issue caused mainly by too many toxins floating throughout the body.

As already mentioned, oxygen-free radicals, highly reactive molecules produced by macrophages and other inflammatory cells, destroy just about anything that comes across their path. They particularly like your DNA! Damaged DNA on the road to destruction allows the mutation process to begin and encourages genes to change their expression relative to aging and disease.

Toxins change your genetic clock, too. The aging process is profoundly accelerated by DNA changes and cellular inflammation. Today, the only biological clock we know of is supported by our telomere, the end-tails of a DNA strand. Upon conception, we carry 15,000 bases of telomeres. By the time we are born, these are reduced to 10,000 base pairs... and we die with only 5,000! Given the fact that the function of telomeres is to protect our DNA, and the fact that every time our cells divide the telomeres become shorter, you can be sure that this mechanism serves to accelerate the aging process. This is the true reason for aging! The wrinkles on your face exist, at least partially, due to cellular toxicity and an internal, imbalanced terrain. If you truly want to look and feel younger, you have to remove the toxins from your cells. Once the body is able to repair its damaged DNA, it can reproduce new cells that express and live a life-affirming and youthful vitality. Then, your cells will dance again!

In the January 2010 volume of the *New Science of Health* it states: "Inflammation seems to underlie not senescence (deterioration with age) but all the chronic illness that often come along with diabetes, atherosclerosis, Alzheimer's, heart attack, cognitive function decline, premature aging and even cancer to an extent."

If you do not have efficient cellular energy production, the body will have a tendency to retain toxins because it simply does not have the cellular fire to burn them up, chemically alter them, or facilitate its required detoxification processes. Of course, many other aspects can lead to inflammation, like pain, a weakened immune system with free-radical pathology, hormone resistance, DNA damage, or to an inability to detox, but it all results in the same problem over and over again: the lack of cellular energy! Stepping away from the biochemical terms, all you need to remember is that free radicals cause inflammation and inflammation causes free radicals. This is the cause and effect scenario that can tip the body into changed cellular behavior and autoimmune conditions. This toxic and harmful inner environment is the very reason for your erratic cellular behavior or illness.

Coming back to our daily diet, common allergens like casein and gluten (proteins found in dairy and wheat) are quick to spark the inflammatory cascade. Anyone suffering from celiac disease knows how inflammatory wheat can be. Foods high in trans fats accelerate LDL levels, the "bad" cholesterol, which feeds inflammation in the arteries. So the first step to cool the fires within on a cellular level has to start with a diet filled with plenty of essential fatty acids, high-quality oils, low protein, and complex carbohydrates added to an abundance of fresh, organic vegetables and fruits. Your food is the real key to chronic inflammation!

My ancestors seldom experienced chronic inflammation or even chronic diseases; in fact when I think back to my childhood I can't recall such things discussed. The diet of my parents and grandparents existed of foods taken directly from the farmer's field without any chemically synthesized compounds or health-altering toxins. I clearly remember early morning walks to the local farmer, holding my dented Milchkanne (milk jug), on my way to collect fresh cow's milk and eggs, produced freshly each day. This milk was clean and rich in superb nutrients, and far from the chemical produced combination of protein and sugar today.

Commercial dairy cows are fed an unnatural diet of grains that produces excessive omega-6 fats. If you are allergic to dairy, as many are, this allergic reaction feeds chronic inflammation. Supermarket beef generally comes from cattle fed with the same unnatural diet of grains that includes hormone residues, steroids, and antibiotics. Not only are these products unnecessary, they're bad for us! And remember, meat is acid, which causes inflammation. It is time to break the habit of consuming acids foods in general, like coffee and sodas. Did you know that sodas contain phosphoric acid, a major contributor to the development of osteoporosis?

When I was young, labeling food was a nonexistent practice, as we all knew where our food came from. We knew the farmer and his family, and we cherished his tireless dedication in providing us with his fresh and nutritious products. When I was nine years old, for one long beautiful year I lived with a farmer's family, tending the animals and walking through the fields at sunrise. I collected potatoes from the Earth's soil, piled up hay, and welcomed the birth of each calf born to their cows. We all smelled of farm, and our hands showed the daily contact with the dark and rich soil, yet that year is one of the fondest and vibrant memories of my young life.

The best way to protect yourself from chronic cellular inflammation focuses on your daily nutrition. Food articles like white flour, bagels, cookies, cereal, sweets, crackers, pizza, grains, high-fat meats, sugar, fast food, and snack foods like potato chips, pretzels, and corn chips all carry pro-inflammatory factors and cause a surge in insulin, which triggers an inflammatory response in the body.

With a daily diet rich in fresh, organic vegetables and a balanced ratio of omega fatty acids you can tone down this reaction. Add plenty of antioxidants and you protect your body from the inflammatory effects of free radicals. Start your day with wild blueberries and goji berries, chia and acacia seeds and add more natural vitamin C in the form of guava, bell peppers, oranges, grapefruit, strawberries, pineapple, kohlrabi, papayas, lemons, broccoli, kale, Brussels sprouts, kidney beans, kiwi, cantaloupe, cauliflower, mangos, and mustard greens. A diverse selection of your chosen vegetables and fruits is the key here!

And remember, good fats are absolutely necessary as part of a nutritious diet because they inhibit a negative immune response and cleanse and lubricate the body. We need fats, as they provide the necessary building blocks for cell membranes and a variety of hormones and hormone-like substances that the body cannot produce alone. Research also educates us on the fact that people on low-fat diets typically suffer from symptoms of depression, fatigue, anxiety, mood swings, hypoglycemia, insulin resistance, constant and insatiable hunger, gall bladder problems, hormonal imbalances, dry and brittle hair, and skin prone to wrinkles.

Dr. Dwight Lundell tells us, "The injury and inflammation in our blood vessels is caused by the low-fat diet recommended for years by mainstream medicine."

As we follow this trend, a diet low in fat and high in polyunsaturated fats (fats that contain more than one double chain of carbon atoms), we literally instigate repeated injury to our blood vessels, causing chronic inflammation leading to heart disease, stroke, diabetes, and obesity.

In the 1940s, researchers thought they'd found a strong correlation between cancer and the consumption of fat. However, at that time, scientists did not make a distinction between hydrogenated, or trans fats (fats in which hydrogen has been added to the oil, turning the liquid oil into a solid block of fat), and saturated fats (referring to the number of hydrogen bonds in the fatty acid molecule). Altered partially hydrogenated fats, made from vegetable oils, block utilization of essential fatty acids, or good fats, lead to sexual dysfunction, increased blood cholesterol, and paralysis of the immune system. The consumption of hydrogenated fats is associated with very serious diseases including cancer, atherosclerosis, diabetes, obesity, immune system dysfunction, low-birth-weight babies, birth defects, difficulty in breast milk production, and problems with bones and tendons.

A daily input of omega-3 oil is therefore an important part of an anti-inflammatory diet, as it forms the building blocks of a number of anti-inflammatory compounds in the body. Countless studies have shown that omega-3s can help prevent heart attacks and sudden cardiac death by preventing arrhythmia (an irregular heartbeat) by making the blood less likely to clot in the arteries. This improves the balance of good and bad cholesterol and limits the dreaded inflammatory process. Today, our modern diet is generally deficient in these essential oils. As already mentioned, the ratio of omega-3 to omega-6 has been shifting disappointingly over the last few decades.

My parents and grandparents were still consuming a balanced ratio of equal proportions of omega-3 omega-6 oils. Our current chosen fast-lifestyle diet typically injects us with 20 times more omega-6 than omega-3 oils. This just can't be healthy for any human! Simply by eliminating your supermarket margarine and reintroducing your good old pure butter, you will create a healthier balance of fat in your body. (Please also refer to the chapter: The Essentials for your Body to Move: The Best Quality Oils.)

The New World of changing paradigms demands the return to a healthy and sustainable attitude to life, from the relationship to the body to the planet! We are now encouraged, invited, and firmly asked, all at the same time, to re-create an intimate co-creative connection to Earth in a new and peaceful revolutionary way, a connection that not only sustains and nurtures our immediate lives but those of many future generations. The wisdom of the body is limitless and is more than our living instrument alone.

༄

So far, I have mainly concentrated on the imbalanced and faulty nutrition that enhances cellular inflammatory processes. Yet, we all know that the body reacts to stress as well, and that stress, whether based on psychological or biological issues, stimulates and ignites movement. Panic, anxiety, daily financial worries, and relationship heartaches create an extra burden on the adrenal glands, responsible for the "fight or flight response." When faced with this feeling of anxiety, the adrenals produce a steroid hormone called cortisol that directly influences insulin levels and the metabolism and adds to chronic inflammation and an over-stressed immune system. Coping with persistent stress takes a real toll on the immune system, the adrenals, and the nervous system.

Most infections lead to inflammatory conditions of one kind or another. Any physical condition based on inflammation is expressed in medical language with "itis" at the end, such as hepatitis, diverticulitis, cystitis, and so on. On a metaphysical level, inflammation is viewed as an internal conflict or warlike in character.

Inflammatory processes in the body march with this war-like frequency. Initially, this destructive nature is played out through battles of external stimuli, like bacteria and viruses, and witnessed as the defending immune system responds with symptoms of heat, fever, and swelling. When the condition settles in to take on a more chronic nature, we can easily observe it in the afflicted individual's mental and emotional personality as well. The inner struggle to overcome the initial trigger manifests itself in ongoing emotional "hot flames" accompanied by frustration, anger, rage, and violence. And we are the witnesses of or the recipients of their angry eruptions and explosive outbursts. The external ongoing quarrel with the spouse might be the manifestation of an internal tooth abscess brought about by an untreated toothache. A burning stomach ulcer, a clear indication of an inflamed gut, often means something is literally eating and burning away at the person.

To truly heal means to be willing to touch and experience our inner wounds and accompanying belief systems. Only then, can we recognize the magical connection between our physical symptoms and our thought patterns. Every infection within the body is given birth from a mental or emotional conflict that takes on a physical form. Any resistance to avoid resolution at the psychological level ultimately leads to chronic inflammation within the cells, tissues, and organs. In the bigger picture, it is easier to meet the smoldering, inner conflict by becoming conscious of a dance that has lost its rhythm within, the inner voices of polarity, and any external symptoms than become the victim of such an ongoing personal war.

Thorwald Dethlefsen and Rüdiger Dahlke state: "Those of us who are unwilling to open our consciousness to conflicts that might irritate us are forced to open our bodies to irritations instead. Then, the disease-agents take up residence in particular weak points within the body, the points of least resistance."

During the course of our lives, we cannot escape irritation in itself, as each and every day is filled with new and challenging situations. We often impulsively react to an unpleasant presented situation, however, rather than meet it with a contemplated response. There is nothing wrong in exploding sometimes or venting your anger and frustration, particularly if you strongly feel about some injustice. Yet it is often beneficial to see all your emotions as fleeting sensations and allow them

Core Body

pass by your eyes like the scenes of a movie. Letting them come and go without being personally involved in or identifying with them helps create movement and energetic flow rather than congestion or cellular inflammation. Once the pain inflames or your body gets sick all your attention will be directed to the physical symptom, diverting your mental and emotional consciousness from its place of resolution.

Daily mental, physical, and emotional irritations are a part of life. As part of the circle of life, irritation should serve us as a reminder to continue to pursue our evolutionary path of truth and beauty more deeply. As soon as you become aware of the level on which the annoyance occurs, you have already broken the chain of perpetuating your habitual reactions. Your contemplative and mindful relationship toward the challenging situation will keep it more in proportion and result in a mature and clear response.

Let's have a look at what happens when we are unable to resolve the agonizing inner conflict on the physical level. In this case, the situation resembles more of a civil war, where two tribes are living in constant disagreement and battle. Inside the body the stimuli, or disease agents, and the defending immune system catalyze this war, as they are now locked in a lifelong battle. In medical terms, this situation is called autoimmune disease. Nobody wins here. The amount of collateral damage is gruesome in its enormity . . . I would suggest far beyond human comprehension. Blood count panels might show permanently raised lymphatic markers, granulocytes, and antibodies, slightly higher blood sedimentation, and perhaps a marginally raised temperature. This constant warring demands the spending of cellular energy to a degree that is sure to leave the individual exhausted—mentally, emotionally, and physically depleted of all ability to resolve this inner turmoil. If he fails to get well and is unable to figure out what is really wrong, he might get depressed. Guaranteed countless and frustrating doctor visits and examinations will fail to produce an accurate diagnosis of the slowly depleting state of health, by then labeled as "Syndrome X," symptoms of unknown origin. The body and the individual have taken the position of an ongoing compromise with no peace or resolution in sight.

Core Body

It is written that Jesus once said: "I wish you were hot or cold. But because you are lukewarm, and neither hot nor cold, I will spew you out of my mouth."

Any compromise based on resignation to the conflict consequently results in stagnation and congestion, like a traffic jam blocking the road. Being bold enough to take the courageous step to make a clear decision in a forward direction, however, can resume the flow and energetic movement. Sometimes decisions are not easy to make because they leave scars and instigate the initial heightening of emotional or physical pain, yet such decisions often ultimately lead to a window of new possibilities.

When I was presented with the situation where I gave my consent to three abdominal surgeries, each three to five months apart, I knew very well that the journey in front of me would be rocky, painful, and stressful. Yet, I also knew that one day I would see the light at the end of that dark tunnel, and that I would arrive at a new spiritual platform enabling me to embrace life with joy and love. This newfound place would be completely different from the one I had left and would not be comparable to anything related to my past. I knew each surgery, each knife cut, and each removal of an organ would bring me closer to the door of liberation.

The loss of organs and scars of this medical intervention caused a turning point in my life, influencing my relationship toward my womanhood, my loved ones, and how I felt about revering and deeply honoring myself. Today, looking back, this experience is what shaped my entire outlook. Since then, literally everything and everybody who wasn't in resonance with honoring and respecting me has slowly but surely faded out of my life. Today, I deeply cherish the experience of this once difficult time.

In my clinical practice, I have seen that even patients with the most severe degenerating symptoms who have gone through the journey of a debilitating illness like cancer usually emerge as spiritually transformed beings because they have consciously evolved into their be-souled Selves. Healing journeys are the journey to our own sanctity.

Core Body

Whatever goes on in the body is experienced in our consciousness as well. To bathe in the sacredness of your Self, do not try to solve your problems in the physical realm alone or to fight a battle only with your body; rather, strive to face and resolve your conflicts on the psychic level first. Wherever there is resistance to change, there is a lack of love. Next time you experience a simple infection or chronic inflammation in your body, ask yourself: What conflict am I failing to see? Who or which situation inflames me? And what can I do to meet the smoldering fire within? Just dare to ask and you will get the answers. In this world of external and internal inflammatory wars, let's usher in a new paradigm of health, based on courage, determination, willingness, and an unwavering self-love that fuels the entire spectrum of our lives.

❧

Let's pause for a moment and take a deep breath. You have taken in a lot of information as you courageously feel and deeply explore your body during your blindfolded dance. Let the dance now come to its close, stand firm and still wherever you are ... and breathe. With each inspiration and expiration watch your breath relax into a sweet and flowing rhythm. Now, gently remove your blindfold, open your eyes, and receive your immediate surroundings with a sense of awe, wonder, and freshness.

You have just emerged from previously uncharted territories and have seen interior images of your body that do not look like the previous, familiar, experiences of yourself and your body-awareness. How do you feel now, having intimately connected with your body? Observe and recognize the nature of your feelings after having journeyed into the depth of yourself. Is there fear? Do you feel a sense of awe and amazement? Accept it all, whatever the present moment contains. Always flow and work with it, not against it. Your next dance is already waiting for you ....

The rhythm of flowing connects us to the flow of our individual energy, our base current. In flowing there are no separations or distinctions between things.

—Gabrielle Roth

Cleansing the Cells to Dance Wild and Free

> The greatest adventure is not going to the moon, the greatest adventure is going to your own innermost core.
>
> —Osho

Ever allowed yourself to dance wild and free without thinking or controlling your dance, a dance without "you" involved? The dancer becomes one with the dance by losing himself and disappearing into the dance. In my early twenties, when I was living on the ashram in India, Osho's teachings encouraged the total immersion of mind, body, and soul through body movements and dance. All different kinds of meditation techniques were based on the radical self-love of accepting and befriending one's body in a revolutionary way, a way that at that time had never before been taught. This place in India stood as the beacon of a living laboratory where eastern and western spiritual techniques and advanced psychotherapy all came together under one roof.

At dawn, we entered the human shell deeply by shaking and moving our bodies to the rising sun. In the evening we danced freely to the setting sun. Each dance brought us one step closer to our freedom and peace. There, I learned to dance wild and free. There, I allowed my soul to be wild and free.

Core Body

Choose a place with a lot of open space and set your intention to completely let go and dance your heart out. Make noises, laugh, sing, cry... whatever your body wants to do, follow it. And, by God, enjoy this dance of your ecstatic wildness. Become your own liberator, a free and sovereign individual. Though you are still locked inside yourself, you are now ready to be freed from your conditioned shackles. Let go, let go, and let go! Once you enter into this boundless and liberated space, your life will never be the same again.

Your body is kindly asking you to take the plunge and reclaim total responsibility in freeing its existence from all accumulated toxins. The most successful and effective way to achieve this goal is to embrace the best cutting-edge natural detoxification program. I am not talking about going to a rehab center that cleans the body from alcohol or drug excess. I am talking about an in-depth, totally transformative journey on the mental, emotional, and physical levels to rid the body of acquired and metabolic toxins by eliminating and breaking destructive and degenerative patterns. I am talking about a detoxification program that is able to meet the dangerous chemical pollution currently, fiercely, penetrating our bodies.

Detoxification is a natural key body function that involves the elimination of metabolic waste: the body's own produced waste and other toxins via the eliminatory organs—the skin, the kidneys, and especially the liver. As much as 80% of all physical chemical processes involve detoxification activities. This comes as no surprise since and modern living has led to an increased exposure of alarming toxic accumulation of a degree never seen before. Next to the toxic by-products of our own metabolism, we are faced with the onslaught of those external incoming toxins.

Particularly over the last three to five years, volatile and disruptive toxins have altered every natural practitioner's viewpoint regarding the scope and depth of a truly successful detoxification program. I well remember the days when alternative medicine practitioners offered (and still continue to offer) the simple spring liver cleanse of lemon juice, garlic, ginger, and olive oil, or simple colon and kidney cleanses. In my clinical practice, these days are over, truly over! Events like the enormous BP oceanic oil spill and the recent nuclear meltdown in Fukushima, Japan, in March 2011, expose us to new neurodegenerative pesticides, herbicides, and radioactive elements that deeply penetrate and settle into the interior of our bodies. The earthquake followed by a catastrophic tsunami set off the worst nuclear accident since Chernobyl, sending three reactor cores into meltdown and causing massive radiation leaks. In the UK, *The Guardian* published an article in March 2012 in which it was confirmed that the Fukushima reactor showed radiation levels much higher than previously reported. In fact, according to the latest examination of the nuclear plant, the damage caused by this disaster is so severe that cleanup phases are expected to take decades. You may not see with your actual eyes or smell the present radioactive pollution slowly spreading over the entire globe, but it clearly exists as evidenced by the Japanese government's recent estimate that the amount of radioactive Caesium-137 released by the Fukushima nuclear disaster thus far is equal to that of 168 Hiroshima bombs (2011)!

Along with these new environmental life-changing forces, our children and future generations are being bombarded with mercury, aluminum, and formaldehyde exposure, all chemical compounds that are chosen as binding and preservative materials in common vaccines, and are now bearing the brunt of humanity's deliberate ignorance.

Over the last five years, it is no coincidence that I am seeing more and more autistic children walking through my practice, Medica Nova. Autism now affects 1 in 66 children; 1 in 54 boys! The prevalence of autism is growing by the year, and more children will be diagnosed with autism this year alone than with AIDS, diabetes, and cancer combined. Autism is the fastest-growing serious developmental disability in the U.S., costing the nation $126 billion per year. Yet this debilitating state of health receives less than 5% of the research funding of many less prevalent childhood diseases. (For further information and help regarding holistic treatments for autism, refer to cases and research material of Tinus Smits, a Dutch homeopath who has gifted humanity with his groundbreaking work regarding homeopathy and autism, at tinussmits.com.)

Core Body

Most of my cases are related to vaccination damage, either directly or indirectly linked to the DPT or MMR inoculations. Anybody with some common sense—no medical expertise is required—would have to ask himself how 49 doses of 14 mandated vaccinations filled with chemical toxins injected before the age of six could not have adverse reactions in an otherwise perfectly healthy but vulnerable child?

For a brief moment, step aside and listen to your primal instinct and common sense. Then you will know the answer! Due to this new palette of environmental toxins penetrating deeper into the body and crossing the blood-brain barrier after reintroduction to the blood and lymphatic channels for elimination, common detoxification programs cannot possibly be as effective as they once were.

Detoxing the body has always played a fundamental role in natural and holistic medicine. Cleansing programs have played a part of man's rituals for health and well-being as far back as 1800 BC. Cleanses and detox diets have long been used in Eastern cultures as a way to maintain optimal health and prevent disease. Ayurvedic medicine also offers many helpful cleansing and rejuvenation treatments.

In whatever form, however, as the world changes, so must our health programs. Even if you could live in a pristine environment and consume only organic, fresh food, you will still be affected by some manner of toxic onslaught. I am blessed to live in one of the most beautiful landscapes of the Southwest of North America. I am surrounded with mountains, clear water, and a blue sky, and immersed in an authentic Native American culture. Yet, come January each year, the sky is plastered with the crisscrossed white lines produced by chemtrails. By February each year, more and more people in my area have begun experiencing seasonal allergies, despite the ground and mountains that are still covered in snow. These new health threats come from all directions: from the thinning ozone layer, ionizing and electromagnetic radiation, environmental chemicals, radioactive air-born particles, and genetically-modified (GM) foods, to fossil fuels and xenobiotic molecules in plastics and cosmetics.

While the alive and dynamic system that is your body is trying very hard to optimize your health, in its core lives a toxic entity, like an energetic tapeworm. A tapeworm injects a chemical into its host that makes it crave things that are good for the tapeworm, but very bad for the host. In this case, we are the hosts—and we are hosting energetic parasites that manipulate and energize themselves at the expense of our well-being! The same principle playing out in the world's environmental and human crisis is playing out in the disease-creating process in our bodies. Today, genetically engineered foods provide an even more significant threat than pesticides and herbicides to our worldwide ecosystems.

John Hagelin, an award-winning quantum physicist has said, "When genetic engineers disregard the genetic boundaries set in place by natural law, they run the risk of destroying our genetic encyclopedia, compromising the richness of our biodiversity, creating a genetic soup. What this means for the future of our ecosystem, no one knows."

And Dr. John Fagan, internationally recognized molecular biologist and former genetic engineer admonishes, "We are living today in a very delicate time, one that is reminiscent of the birth of the nuclear era, when mankind stood on the threshold of a new technology. No one knew that nuclear power would bring us to the brink of annihilation or fill our planet with highly toxic radioactive waste. We are so excited by the power of a new discovery that we leaped ahead blindly and without caution. Today, the situation with genetic engineering is perhaps even more grave because this technology acts on the very blueprint of life itself."

Rather than condemning and blaming the state of health in the population on our planet's environmental and man-made disasters or on the dreaded corporate pharmaceutical monopolies, we are all asked to rise to the challenge. Let us meet this dilemma with new, innovative, and excellent natural treatments so that we, as a new species, can change this outlived paradigm poisoning the world and our bodies. Today, a good detoxification program becomes one of the most important health regimes for the body. You can't do without it anymore!

Anyone who wants to protect his health, rebuild his health, and maintain his optimal health must detoxify his body. Chronic degenerative diseases in particular are almost impossible to meet effectively without a clear and thorough cleansing plan that addresses such a wide scope of toxins that weaken the body's defenses and make us more susceptible to disease and stress.

No one is exempt from the need for a deep cleansing program. Once a year is advocated, but for people with serious health issues, I recommend a detoxification program every six months, as the body will benefit from releasing accumulated toxins more often. Others who experience serious toxicity issues with a deep-seated illness might even think about engaging in a yearlong support program.

There are many options available: The Master Cleanse, juice fasting, smoothies, pure water fasting, commercial cleanse programs (available at your health food shop), raw food detox diets, Ayurvedic and rejuvenation protocols (like Panchakarma), elimination, candida, macrobiotic, and digestive cleanses. These detox diets can be followed for 3 to 7 days or longer. Some programs are not as restrictive as juice fasts or the Master Cleanse, and most people are usually able to follow them while continuing with their everyday lives. Fasting, on the other hand, which can cause nausea, headaches, skin rashes, diarrhea, bad breath, or a Herxheimer's reaction (a short-term "healing crisis"), often has the best results when one can take the time to go on retreat or take a break from the daily routine. Whichever detox program you undertake, it is always recommended to do it with the support of an experienced healthcare practitioner who can tailor the program to your individual needs.

Normally, detox diets eliminate potential dietary allergens, dietary toxins and chemicals (such as pesticide residues), and foods that have an inflammatory effect on the body. Of course, processed foods are completely avoided during this time. There is an emphasis on reducing acidity and mucus in the body in order to create a more alkaline environment.

Often people make a practice of fasting one day a week to allow their bodies time to cleanse and recover. Others choose natural supplementation programs. Unfortunately, most people never even contemplate the idea of a periodic detox program. Reasons include: I don't have the money," "I don't have the time," "I am too sensitive to take so many supplements" (which simply means this person is very toxic already!) and "I'm too busy and travel too much to do anything like that!"

Core Body

Yet when the body falls ill, these are the people who make time to see a physician or check into the nearest hospital.

Envision the following scenario. You have just woken up. With your cup of coffee in your hand you look out your living room window to find your car sitting right on the road. Somebody has sliced into four tires of your car during the night! What do you do? I am sure that without hesitation you would buy four new tires, as you need your car to move through your life. The same principle applies to your health, which needs you as an active participant in the creation of your well-functioning body. Do not sit around and expect the body to do it all for you. You are an intimate part of this journey and only with your conscious participation will you see and feel the necessary changes. With a well-designed detoxification program undertaken at least once a year, you will not only prevent future diseases, but the quality of your life will remarkably improve in all areas from wealth to spirituality.

Most suggested detox cleanses, like the ones mentioned above, are limited by today's standards. They belong to an old model of cleansing the body. These treatment protocols, based on singular approaches like raw food diets, organic juice therapies, bowel cleanses, lymphatic drainage massages, infrared saunas, and liver flushes are still important and valid therapies, but do not address the toxicity of the extra-cellular and interior terrain of the cells. That is why in this chapter I introduce you to the most scientifically advanced detoxification program, designed for this changing New World. The new model of detoxification includes all the benefits of the old therapies with our added new understanding of cellular biology. This new model of understanding and implementing the stages of effective cellular cleansing will certainly be part of the new medicine and the entry point into the New World.

Detoxification is a special time and can be a spiritual awakening. Old processes are cast away. Deep-seated disturbances come to the surface to be addressed and discarded. The removal of heavy metals and toxins raises the body's vibratory rate. It's the necessary step before renewal. —Dr. Jack Tips

Core Body

Benefits of Detoxing and Re-building the Body

PHYSICAL BENEFITS

The first time I completed a detoxification program I felt a distinct sense of a deep rejuvenation within my body and all organs. Stored-up toxins, dormant for months and years, were released and eliminated. My liver felt happy and soft again, and I experienced a palpable ease that traveled throughout my entire digestive system. My liver, colon, stomach, kidneys, neuroendocrine system, and mental faculties, along with all the other parts of my body, began to work more effectively. My life became more productive and certainly more creative.

After a detox, people often report feeling lighter and experiencing more energy during their workouts and daily chores. As the program clears away heavy metals, stored chemicals, biofilms, and free radicals, the body's immune system becomes stronger and more resilient to external stimuli like colds and flu. The blood is cleansed, supporting circulation throughout the entire body—the prime factor for vitality and longevity. Life feels so much better. Life feels good again!

MENTAL BENEFITS

Toxins and free radicals can affect brain function. Sleep problems, lack of concentration, learning difficulties, lack of memory, general brain fog, and chronic exhaustion are all indicators of a congested brain. After detoxification, people often experience a clarity and sharpness of their mental faculties that surprises them. Even during challenging and emotional times, they find themselves capable of making more responsible and clear distinctions regarding their life circumstances. This newly regained mental power is applicable in all areas of their lives: personal relationships, clearing away cluttered or unresolved issues, developing creative projects . . . the list goes on. Though I have learned to expect such results, the phenomenon is always a welcome surprise as it brings with it a sudden spontaneity and clarity that I deeply cherish.

LIFESTYLE CHANGES

As you journey through the cleansing process feeling better and healthier by the day, you naturally want to let go of certain habitual behaviors, like tobacco, alcohol, and recreational drugs. You may find you want to change your diet, introduce an exercise regime into your daily schedule, or join a yoga class. This new relationship to life will gradually and with ease emerge from the very core of your being. You will feel a strong urge birthed from deep inside of you to participate in your very own life-changing event rather than blindly accepting mainstream trends imposed by those expecting you to change. In this very moment, you want to change, as you want to maintain this newfound sense of vibrancy. You want to stay healthy.

To embrace a detoxification program is a dance you will never forget!

The Systemic Detoxification Program for the New World

First let's look at some common symptoms that could indicate you may need a detox cleanse. If you experience ongoing headaches, migraines, depression, fatigue and low energy, hormone problems, menstrual and reproductive problems, trouble sleeping, muscle pain, joint stiffness and pain, stomach pain, acid reflux, irritable bowel syndrome, short-term memory loss, muscle twitching, chronic degenerative diseases, autoimmune diseases, skin eruptions, and/or difficulty losing weight despite exercise and diet, there is no doubt you are in need of a cleansing regime.

Any successful detoxification program will target the liver, with its Healing Triad (mentioned in the chapter "Toxicity Dances Through the Body"). Dr. A Stuart Wheelwright strongly emphasizes that true healing relies on a well-functioning liver triad comprised of the liver, stomach, and colon. When food is poorly digested and ferments the resultant toxins impact the liver's ability to function to capacity. Since the overburdened liver cannot conduct its detoxification process adequately, it passes the buck (filled with toxins) to the kidneys, the next organ in line.

Build the liver's vitality, and the liver will detoxify the body according to the body's inherent detoxification pathways. —A. S. "Doc" Wheelwright

Why is it absolutely necessary to support the liver from the onset of any detoxification program? To recap, the liver is the single most important organ in the body—even more important than the heart, due to its countless life-maintaining functions. The body's main natural detoxifier has a huge effect not only on our physical health and longevity through its removal of poisons and metabolic waste products, but also on our mental and emotional states. The liver produces 50,000 enzymatic systems that govern metabolic activity and neutralize harmful substances. It is not only one of our largest organs in the human body, but our central organ.

The liver has two detoxification pathways: Phase One and Phase Two. Each phase requires the work of different nutrients. During Phase One, a toxic chemical is altered into a less harmful one, resulting in the formation of free radicals. Sufficient numbers of antioxidants are required to quench the activity of the free radicals. Without sufficient amounts, the free radicals have free reign to damage the liver cells. In Phase Two, a toxic chemical is made water-soluble by the additional substance that moves it out of the body through the colon or kidneys.

The liver is also the primary drainage system for the body, which deals with toxins of high molecular weight, like heavy metals. A sluggish liver, one that functions poorly, will express itself as some kind of intolerance. This means your body will negatively react even to the slightest consumption of alcohol, for instance, or foods that are rich and fatty. If you experience nausea, bloating after meals with overall digestive problems, constipation, or irritability, you can almost be certain that your liver needs extra help. Improving your liver function will also help you manage your weight, as the body holds onto liquids (a condition referred to as "water retention") or onto fat, which serves as a storage unit of excess toxins. Hormonal problems are not only due to hormonal changes as one might assume, but are often the cause of liver imbalances as well. The common Premenstrual Syndrome (PMS) that includes symptoms of moodiness from crying to angry outbursts occurs when the liver is not able to break down the hormones efficiently and an imbalance or accumulation of estrogen results.

As you can see, once the liver is unable to handle the initial detoxification process on its own, as it is meant to do, all the other organs and bodily systems can be exposed to the toxicity. Needless to say, during a cleanse it is not advisable to not overburden the body with extra toxic substances like alcohol, excessive sugar, or caffeine.

The body has different ways to rid itself of accumulated toxins. The gallbladder moves toxins into the intestines; the kidneys excrete toxins via urination; the lungs expel toxins during exhalation; the skin sweats out excess toxicity; the lachrymal ducts cry out toxic tears; the sinuses drain their channels of mucus; the menstrual period causes bleeding and the releasing of fibrous tissue; the colon excretes fecal matter; the ears produce wax; and the hair releases its own load of toxicity as it grows. The entire body is in a constant spring-cleaning process, provided the exit channels are clean and uncongested.

Imagine the liver as the main port where all the ships carrying their large freights dock. Here the arriving ships are cleared of their cargo, maintained, and set off on their next journey. Without this central port, there is no efficient transport system of goods and livestock to support the world market. The liver acts as a central port within the body, providing and stabilizing the vital nutrients and processes for its well-being.

I highly recommend my favorite detoxification program, described below, to all my patients. It is safe, comprehensive, and effective.

Core Body

The Three Phases of the Systemic Detoxification Program

PHASE ONE

My most recommended detoxification program is called The Ultimate Whole-Body Cleanse For Radiant Health. This cleanse consists of three phases, each covering 20 to 30 days, depending on the patient's sensitivity and health status. Phase One concentrates on a deep cleanse of the Healing Triad of liver, left liver lobe, gallbladder, stomach, and colon. Some individuals experience a slight headache during this initial process, but most sail through without any problem.

I highly recommend adding a daily detox bath during this first phase. Soak yourself in a bathtub filled with hot water and add 2 lb. of sea salt, Epson salt (magnesium sulfate) or Celtic salt, and 2 lb. of baking soda. Soak for 30 minutes while you drink some lemon water. Your body may start to sweat, which is a great sign. Let it happen! This bath is activating your skin to release more toxins. You can also brush your skin with a natural scrubbing sponge, called a loofah, or Luffa, which activates your lymphatic system to excrete more toxins via your skin. Always make sure your brush movements lead toward, not away, from your heart.

PHASE TWO

Most commercial cleanses stop right here! Although they all have some beneficial effect on the liver, stomach, colon, and kidneys, most do not go further into the interior of the body. As a healthcare practitioner, I am personally invested in exploring the depths and unchartered territories of the body and self. That is why the second phase of this superb detoxification program works on the extra-cellular matrix (ECM), the very part that is situated between the cells or collagen. This is where toxins are stored when the regular detoxification processes of the liver, gall bladder, kidneys, and lungs have not been able to handle the extra workload. On this extra-cellular level, toxins build up inside fat cells, called adipose cells, and are deposited in the fibrous collagen that connects and supports other bodily tissues such as skin, bone, tendons, muscles, and cartilage. Once the toxins settle in the fat cells, the pH of the body's tissues alters. This situation creates an environment susceptible to pathogens, in particular, biofilms or biomasses. It is only a matter of time before one's general health status is negatively influenced.

In my experience, allopathic medicine never talks about these detrimental elements called biofilms. Biofilms are aggregates of microorganisms, like the sacs of slime barrier that shield dangerous spirochetes and other bacteria, fungus, and viruses from the immune system. In order to protect itself from these breeding nests and to continue to function at its optimal level, the body creates sealed pockets of toxicity. But there is a price to pay! Though "sealed," these packets are only lying dormant. Like time bombs, they can go off at any time and deplete your immune system and overall health. Once these biofilms break open, the spill of collected and breeding toxins resembles an oil spill in the ocean.

A diet based on trans-fats in the form of starches like potato chips and donuts contributes to the development of biofilms in the extracellular matrix. Incorporating this important second phase of the detox program is especially necessary for anybody who suffers from chronic candida or fungal infections.

Another important factor, often overlooked, has to do with the life-depleting danger that exists once the toxins are released into the bloodstream. If poisons fail to be altered by cellular methylation (see Phase Three) or a chelator molecule that binds them and makes them less offensive, they can spill over into the brain and interfere with the neuroendocrine system. This situation brings us to the hormone-producing glands, like the hypothalamus, pituitary, pineal, thyroid, and eventually the adrenal glands, the next ones in line to carry the toxic bucket.

In Phase Two, the cells are provided with extra energy and nutrients that cleanse and prepare the body for Phase Three. That's why it is absolutely necessary in Phase Two to support the hypothalamic/pituitary/pineal axis. The goal is to rectify the dreaded inflammatory processes here, before they start taking over the whole body.

Core Body

Another very important point that has gone unmentioned in the common literature refers to standard weight-loss programs. As toxins are expelled from the extra-cellular matrix, fat cells give up their fat reservoirs with the released stored toxins. These fat-soluble toxins are suddenly freed to swim about in the lymphatic and circulatory systems. This is not a good idea! Now, the pressure is on, as these toxins must be cleared from the body quickly.

You can see why it is so essential to start by cleaning and building a strong and efficient liver to meet the considerable tasks of the detoxification period. If this process cannot be met, heavy metal toxicity appears throughout the body. Just as lead can bond with bones, mercury can cross the blood-brain barrier and Strontium-90 can get into the bone marrow, creating tumors. Not a good idea indeed! Are you appreciating how a detoxification program should be strong enough to back up all the subtle yet important steps during its implementation? This is also the reason why some cleanses result in a Herxheimer's reaction, or healing crisis.

I once had an unpleasant experience with an intravenous chelation therapy of EDTA (ethylenediaminetetraacetic acid) to help remove the heavy metals contaminating my body. Usually this treatment is safe and has been successfully applied all over the world. As soon as the IV started, however, I felt a very uncomfortable pressure at the back of my neck, immediately alarming me that the released toxins were moving into my brain area. I believe that this situation would not have occurred if the therapy had included the appropriate building up of the liver and support of the neuroendocrine system. Please, even if you are offered the best detoxification program on the market, make sure that these important points of information are covered before your embark on any cleansing regime. This aggravation time is unnecessary, often a setback in the healing process, and does not focus on the new model of wholeness.

In Phase Two, the Ultimate-Whole Body Detox Program removes toxins from the extra-cellular terrain, but also clears out the bottleneck toxins, opens more drainage pathways, supports the neuroendocrine system, and continues with the absolutely necessary liver support.

Core Body

PHASE THREE

Ah! And now the icing on the cake! It gets better as we go along. In Phase Three, this comprehensive cleansing program deals with the interior of your cells. Up to this point, no known detoxification program has tackled the issue of looking at the interior world of the cells, which comprise the very core of your body and your Self. The New World ushers in not only a paradigm of new consciousness, but also the unique and transformative marriage among science, medicine, and spirit. The scientific community has finally embarked on research regarding cellular biology and its importance in the creation of most (80%) of all our diseases. Not only are we living through one of the most exciting times in history, but we are also witnessing the fundamental transformation within our bodies to achieve optimal health. And you are part of it!

❧

At this point, the toxins have traveled deep into the interior of the body and settled quite comfortably around the cell membrane, the outer cell wall, or within the cell. This results in interference in the integrity and communication system of the cell membrane and creates common and almost epidemic symptomatologies such as hormone resistance, particularly in women, by interrupting their entire hormonal systems. Excessive menstrual disturbances with alternating moods, either during the years of menses or during perimenopause (the menopausal transition) and menopause are mostly related to a congested liver and toxic overburdened cell membranes.

We can use apples to make this point. Imagine an apple with a wonderful red, shiny skin. If the apple is a product of G. M. Frankenstein Science, it is infused with toxic properties, which affect the outer layer, the skin or membrane, and the apple's interior, leaving it with depleted nutrients. This apple never flourished under natural conditions where it soaked up the sun's rays to be transformed into vital energy. Its own natural, full-cycle growth process never energized it. Conversely, as the membrane of the apple is unable to receive beneficial elements, nutrients located in the interior of the apple are unable to exit through its membrane, serving the immediate environment of the apple. What nutrients there are, located inside the apple, are unable to exit through its impenetrable immediate environment. The symbiosis between the apple (the human) and its environment and communication system has been permanently interrupted.

This scenario can be compared to a communication crisis when telephone cables are down or mobile phone networks are out of service and no one is able to reach anyone else. In the body, all our organs, tissues, and glands are trying to communicate with each other, yet are unable to get their messages across to the messages' receivers. Here, all hormonal systems are affected. Insulin resistance causes diabetes, obesity, and heart disease; glucagon resistance leads to hepatic steatosis, or a fatty liver, and the commonly found thyroid resistance affects the under-functioning thyroid gland (contributing to obesity) as does leptin resistance, the primal cause of obesity today.

But that's not all! Follicle-stimulating hormone resistance leads to ovarian atrophy; luteinizing hormone resistance affects male and female gonadal dysfunction; estrogen resistance causes menstrual and menopausal issues as well as breast and uterus or prostate cancer; progesterone resistance can cause endometriosis, breast tenderness, and irregular menses; and testosterone resistance leads to muscle loss, prostate cancer, and erectile dysfunction. Your under-functioning thyroid may well be healed by looking at these important factors rather than pumping up your body with a lifelong course of a synthetically produced drug.

Did you know that current statistics show that about 15 million people in the U.S. are affected with autoimmune thyroid disease, of which 12.5 million are diagnosed with Hashimoto and 2.5 million with Graves' disease? This means that today most women and men are afflicted with some level of endocrine system imbalance. I can verify this propensity in my own clinical practice, where I see that my patients' degenerative diseases are often birthed by disturbances of the endocrine system. Why? The answer clearly revolves around environmental toxicity and cellular inflammation.

Core Body

Deep-seated toxins are the main cause of inflammation of the cell membrane. I already introduced you to the overall concept of cellular inflammation, yet here these toxins will target the cell membrane, the true brain center of the cell. When the membrane inflames and becomes unable to receive and convert the incoming messages due to its damaged receptors and receptor genes, which are unable to receive vital nutrients for their cell interiors regarding ATP or cellular energy production, it is only a matter of time until the cell prematurely starves or dies from the lack of life-giving energy supply. Scientists today agree that a lack of ATP is the root cause of all diseases. For your cells to live happily-ever-after their membranes must let nutrients and molecules enter their interiors and must allow toxins to exit through their membrane walls.

Detoxification is an absolutely necessary pathway for the body to overcome symptoms, chronic degenerative diseases and autoimmune diseases. No two ways about it. It's got to be done, so let's do it right! – Dr. Jack Tips

During Phase Three of our cleanse, high doses of antioxidants are introduced to protect the cell membrane from a chemical process caused lipid peroxidation. In simple terms, this destructive chemical process called the NO/ONOO Cycle causes havoc and more inflammation to the cell membrane, as does the self-inflicted free radical damage of the cell interior. In order to break such toxic cycles we need our chief antioxidant called glutathione to step forward.

I realize this information is a bit scientific and that you may have to dive deeper into the very depth of your interior to follow along. You may not be all that interested in science or you may feel stretched by so many unfamiliar biochemical terms. But please be reassured that the knowledge presented will all make sense soon.

Now, back to our toxins, which have already deeply disrupted cellular function. Is there nothing we can do to stop this toxic trend? Yes, there is. The good news is that with the help of an in-depth detoxification program our genes can be positively influenced in breaking this downward spiral of self-destruction!

Although inflamed membranes and free radical damage can profoundly affect our DNA and influence our genetics, the path of any degenerative disease can be interrupted. This is where our cellular freedom of choice comes into play! Always be aware that you are the author of your life story and the creator of your lifestyle. You are in control of much of your cellular environment, which deeply affects your genetic make-up.

In the chapter "Inviting Your Illness to the Dance Floor," I already spoke about this brilliant bodily built-in chemical process called "methylation" which will certainly become an invaluable part of the new model of medicine. If we are lacking life-altering "helpers" (called methyl groups, alkyls derived from methane, containing one carbon atom bonded to three hydrogen atoms, or CH_3), however, then we have inadequate resources to sustain the process of methylation for all functions that initiate a gradual or abrupt onset of symptoms and disease. While it's true that genetics plays a role, our genes are not the only culprits that cause illness. In fact, single-gene disorders affect less than 2% of the population. The reality is that most of us come into this world with genes that should enable us to live a healthy life.

Methylation is a mechanism that indirectly influences gene expression, but does not involve a permanent change in DNA expression. It is like a switch that can be turned on or off depending on the incoming information or command. It is also the same inherent switch, for example, that either instigates the growth or inhibits the life of a tumor. DNA methylation is the biological process by which the methyl groups, described above, are added to DNA nucleotides. DNA, or deoxyribonucleic acid, is an important nucleic acid that stores the genetic information for any given organism. Many different types of organisms can undergo DNA methylation, though not always with the same results. In plants, for example, scientists believe that methylation occurs to deactivate genes that could otherwise cause harmful mutations. In fungi, DNA methylation is used to moderate and control the expression of certain genes based on the particular conditions affecting the fungus. Methylation in mammals similarly moderates and inhibits the expression of certain genes, like a dormant illness. Additionally, methylation is involved in the production of chromatin, a protein-DNA complex that makes up the structure of chromosomes.

When these important methyl groups are depleted due to stress, emotional upsets, or chemical imbalances, other bodily functions are reduced, leading to the onset of many diseases, including cancer, lupus, muscular dystrophy, birth defects, and premature aging. This situation also plays a role in the hormone deregulation as well as hormone-related cancers due to the non-removal of toxic estrogen metabolites. We also see more autoimmune diseases caused by the lack of these important methyl groups. By the way, did you know that the National Cancer Institute has stated that at least 60% of cancers originate from environmental causes?

This is why natural supplementation of methyl groups, particularly during a 60 to 90-day systemic detoxification period, is so critical for decreasing toxic environmental influences, including deficient nutrition, stress, and intense emotional phases.

The environment changes the behavior of your cells! This science of understanding the importance of both internal and external environmental influences in conjunction with cutting-edge, newly developed detoxification programs prepared for the New World and its unfolding challenges bridges the way for effective holistic healing even more. Even if you find it difficult to understand the biochemical concepts presented here, you certainly see how your active participation in your well-being and optimal health is absolutely essential for your cellular transformation. The environment you create, in your mind, home, and workplace influences the state of your health, right down to the very core of your cells.

Bruce H. Lipton, author and biologist states: "When methyl groups attach to a gene's DNA, it changes the way regulatory chromosomal proteins bind to the DNA molecule. Methylating DNA can silence or modify gene activity. The malignancies in a significant number of cancer patients are derived from environmentally induced epigenetic alterations and not defective genes."

Our DNA does not control our biology! Our cells behave like miniature mirrors reflecting the way we live. In the very beginning of this book, I introduced you to the fundamental understanding of health relative to its ability to adapt to environmental changes. The same principle relates to the health of our cells. Genes are not able to preprogram a cell or any organism's life because the cell's survival depends on the ability to adjust to an ever-changing environment. This is the meaning of health in the macrocosm and microcosmic terrains.

If you live in an abusive and oppressive relationship your cells will act and behave according to this negative energy field. It doesn't take a rocket scientist to understand that the mind and body will only able to heal if you change the existing environment, either by leaving the abuser or changing the situation. If a person is riddled with rheumatoid arthritis, yet lives in a damp or mold-infested accommodation, even the best natural treatment protocols will only be partially successful, as the permanent and existing cause, the dampness and mold, will continue to affect the recipient. In order to heal, you have to remove the cause of the situation!

Our biological terrain, the body, is shaped to function with all its brilliance or to decay, fueled and defined by mental and emotional stress, physical trauma, nutritional deficiencies, toxic overload, and general constitution, the soil of our individual gardens. Until recently, the belief was that our cellular blueprint (DNA) couldn't be changed, that it was given to us as a fixed protocol at the time of conception.

Life is an ever-changing process, however, never stagnant and in ever-evolving movement. Therefore, we are always intimately involved in the participation of our lives. We are constantly activating or deactivating our DNA by our responsible or less responsible choices during the course of our lives.

You are an active participant in your evolution and not just a carbon copy of a concept from the past. Your conscious choices will affect the cellular blueprint of your present and future health and well-being.

꽃

As we explore the nature and life of a cell, we see that our body's true brain is not necessarily situated in the actual brain matter only, but resides in the cell membranes and in the heart. This thought alone awakens our consciousness to much vaster realms. Furthermore, the cell's inherent intelligence is enhanced by utilizing its outer cell membrane surface more efficiently or by expanding its surface area, resulting in better cell communication. Can you believe that you can have such an amazing effect on your own cellular biology? You, and only you, can flick the switch to either live in optimal and vibrant health or lingering disease!

We understand that proteins are our basic physical building blocks. Only when complementary environmental signals animate these significant building blocks do they want to move—to dance. How does this process really work? The cell membrane carries two types of antennas, one called the receptor protein and the other the effector protein. Receptor proteins provide the cell with an awareness of its surrounding environment, while the effector proteins turn on or off the cell's switches to generate signals that we feel and experience as physical sensations. These sensations directly influence and regulate cellular functions.

The interrelated connection between environment and physical symptoms can be seen in the following case scenario. An asthmatic child, five years of age, lives in an extremely stressful household where the mother suffers from bipolar disorder and the father drowns in chronic alcoholism. The child experiences this stressful environment as pure anxiety, as she never knows when or can prepare herself for her mother's sudden and unpredictable outbursts or her father's emotional and physical abuse when he comes home drunk. In this situation, the receptor proteins attached to this child's cell membranes are constantly registering the nature of the surrounding environment, making her aware of the environment's "frequency," a frequency we might call "danger." The effector proteins flip the switch within those membranes, letting her know it is time to feel that dangerous frequency. In response, the child experiences anxiety, which transpires as the physical constriction of her lungs' airways with resultant asthma attacks and chronic cellular inflammation.

The communication between our environment and our cells might look like an international phone call, spreading over oceans and miles of distance, yet the context of the message stays the same no matter how far it has to travel.

This interplay of turning on or off genetic or behavioral patterns, all of which are situated in our cell membranes, clearly demonstrates the importance of the interrelationship between our physical sensations and our surrounding environment. In other words, how you perceive your life, including the nature of your relationship to your loved ones, friends, and everybody with whom you engage, controls your cellular behavior. As you choose a life fueled with an overall positive perception, your health systematically improves. Contrarily, if you consistently expose yourself to a negative and life-depleting environment, your health is sure to decline. Your life experience can actively influence your genetic blueprint. Think about this for a moment!

Again, what happens within the cell membrane is what causes the interface between environmental signals and proteins acting out their respected behavioral patterns. The cell membrane is like the brain of the cell, making countless decisions fueled by these incoming signals. From the external environment to your interior environment of thoughts, emotions, and cellular levels of toxicity, your cells respond and behave according to their respective incoming frequencies.

༄

As you can see, there are only two sources in the creation of cellular disease: damaged cellular proteins or receptors or distorted incoming signals. The experience of a sudden, unforeseen mental, emotional, or physical trauma along with excessive toxicity within the body can influence the cells to malfunction. Cellular "malfunction" leads to cellular inflammation, with which we are so familiar.

Bruce H. Lipton states: "Each cell's unique set of identity receptors is located on the membrane's outer surface, where they act as antennas, downloading complementary environmental signals. These identity receptors read a signal of self, which does not exist within the cell but comes to it from the external environment. The cell's receptors are not the source of its identity but the vehicle by which the 'self' is downloaded from the environment. This means, my identity, my 'self,' exists in the environment whether my body is here or not."

Might this be the answer to the inquiry regarding the nature of the soul? We will explore this question further in the next chapter, but suffice to say that it all boils down to the same core principle: the way you live your life influences the character of your true self! In the course of a lifetime pain is unavoidable, but suffering is optional!

A thorough detoxification program supports gene expression, which protects against the overwhelming amount of toxins in the environment. Your body and you go hand in hand.

It is not uncommon for a patient to question me about why he has cellular toxicity despite eating an organic and healthy diet. The answer here does not revolve around one's genes and the tendency to attract pathogens, but rather has everything to do with the efficiency of one's inherent detoxification system. Research suggests that our capacity to naturally detoxify our bodies varies from person to person. A study in Hawaii, for example, suggests that people with various backgrounds differ from one another by a nearly 20-fold difference in their ability to detox. The research data suggests that only one-third of the variation is associated to diet itself.

If we continue to overload our bodies with an onslaught of self-inflicted and environmental toxins, it is only a matter of time before the body breaks down and loses its ability to detoxify malignant or degenerative diseases. We have to create a livable and healthier environment that minimizes exposure to these detrimental toxins, as well as cleanse and build up our physical inherent detoxification systems by consuming the highest quality of uncontaminated, fresh and organic foods. In this way, we build a strong and lasting immunity shield ready to meet such challenging circumstances.

THE NEW MODEL OF DETOXIFICATION INCLUDES:
- Complete liver and kidney support
- Digestive Support
- Bowel support

Core Body

- Gall Bladder support
- Complete drainage support
- Extracellular matrix support
- Neuroendocrine support
- A complete anti-aging package
- Antioxidant protection
- Daily nutrition
- ATP/energy production and methylation support
- Cell membrane support

As you can see, simple detoxification programs, available over-the-counter in health food shops or via the Internet, are not be able to meet the complex package of cellular toxicity we currently face. Fortunately, science and spirit have advanced to the degree that we have the finest biochemical minds in the field of life-enhancing detoxification programs providing us the help we need today.

How to Assist the Body During the Detoxification Process

During any detoxification program it is important to consume considerable phytonutrients, organic fruit, vegetables, and fresh herbs, like fresh dandelion leaves, which support the liver in the cleansing process. This is true whether the program is a juice fast, a classic liver cleanse, or a Master Cleanse, but particularly true during the Ultimate-Whole Body Detoxification Program. The diet should also be low in fat and high in fiber. Adding more brightly colored fruits and vegetables, like blueberries, carrots, or beetroot, all rich in antioxidants, helps, too. By increasing your vegetable content, you naturally increase the alkalinity within your body. It has been clinically proven that artichokes maintain a healthy liver by improving bile flow as well as lowering cholesterol, so think about adding some artichokes to your next meal to boost support for this wonderful organ.

Eat lighter meals at more frequent intervals during the day instead of filling yourself with a large plate of food. It is especially important to consume a lighter evening meal, as the liver will have its well-deserved rest during the hours of sleep.

Drink plenty of water. Water aids in the elimination of toxins via the kidneys. On waking or before meals, drink a glass of hot lemon juice to stimulate your liver and digestive tract.

Of course, avoid alcohol, caffeinated products, cigarettes, and recreational drugs, as well as heavily processed food or junk food. Fried foods are a source of free radicals and other harmful substances, all of which force the liver to work harder to process. Make an effort to avoid all bad fats. Saturated fat from meat, dairy, and fat-laden snacks such as crisps and peanuts, for instance, also stress the liver. Liver cirrhosis (scarring of the liver) occurs not only from excess alcohol, but also from excess fat, which damages the liver cells, especially if the diet lacks antioxidants.

Meat should be limited while detoxing due to its high-acid, high-fat, and high-protein content. Toxins also tend to accumulate higher up the food chain, and many meat products contain hormones and antibiotics that have to be broken down by the liver.

Avoid Sugar! Sugar depletes the body of many minerals and interferes with blood sugar control, forcing the liver to manipulate its glycogen stores more than it normally would.

Avoid most common grains during the program. Grains are simply sugar derivatives and the prime cause, next to bad fats, for inflammatory conditions in the body. We are all familiar with the increasing epidemic of gluten intolerance, which is spreading worldwide. Gluten is a protein structure found in most grains. An amazing 30% of the global population is already inflicted—and this number is growing! Initially, people diagnosed with celiac disease were the ones more at risk and affected. But today we are all at risk for experiencing the side effects of industrially produced grains. Wheat and corn are found in almost every processed food today, from soda, chewing gum, spaghetti sauce, and extracts, to soups. Gluten sensitivity and gluten intolerance is strongly linked with attention deficit disorders (ADD/ADHD), hyperactivity, depression, anxiety, and Alzheimer's disease. Most of us focus on gluten as the culprit of most intestinal diseases, yet other molecules in the wheat structure also cause low-level chronic inflammation, ultimately altering cell function and cell membranes. Wheat, as well as spelt and rye, contains high amounts of a molecule called lectin, or wheat germ agglutinin (WGA), which promotes inflammation of the body.

Therefore, it is best to avoid all grains while you lighten the load for the liver to prepare your body to heal and rebuild again. The grains available in our shops today are far removed from the quality of grains from even fifty years ago; certainly from the grains people consumed thousands of years ago. The loaf of bread we buy at the bakery or supermarket has been hybridized, genetically modified, and altered to resist fungal infection by literally soaking it with toxic pesticides. What we are eating may look like a wholesome crispy slice of bread, but more resembles a slice of toxic chemical compounds.

During this special time of cleansing the body, allow yourself ample hours of sleep. Reduce your daily stress by enjoying a relaxing bath at the end of the day. Honor yourself by giving yourself the opportunity to heal. Perhaps listen to your favorite soft music, and then go to bed early. Give yourself the time to relax and rest. Today is today and tomorrow is another day, yet we only have this very moment. This is your life!

This brilliant and Ultimate-Whole Body Detoxification Program, covering all three phases of organ and cellular detoxification and designed by the team at Systemic Formulas, stands at the forefront of all detoxification programs on the market so far. I wholeheartedly offer this program, not just to all my patients, but also to everybody interested in healing from the core. For further information, contact my practice, Medica Nova, at www.medicanova.net.

A periodic systemic detox is essential for optimal health in the 21st century. It enlivens the body's innate vitality to better express optimal health, joy and longevity. And best of all, it helps remove the cause of many "no known cause, no known cure" health concerns. Herein is the dividing line between health and infirmity. —Dr. Jack Tips

Core Body

Congratulations, you did it! I am impressed how your passion to heal from your very core has brought you this far. It takes courage, determination, and perseverance to hold the beacon of true change. After having deeply explored your mind and conditioned belief system, built an intimate relationship with your body, embarked on a new nutritional diet, and deeply transformed the lives of your cells and their present and future generations, you have metamorphosed into a completely new being ready to spread its wings like a newborn butterfly. Don't be shy. Show us your new colors, twirl around, and let yourself be seen. Look at yourself; embrace the newfound you and rejoice in your vibrant state of optimal health. It took a lot of work and countless different dances to arrive at this place of sheer bliss and peace. Your dance is magnificent and deeply inspiring.

In honor of your dedication, let's dance together, you and I, by embracing the next step into your deepest core, your soul.

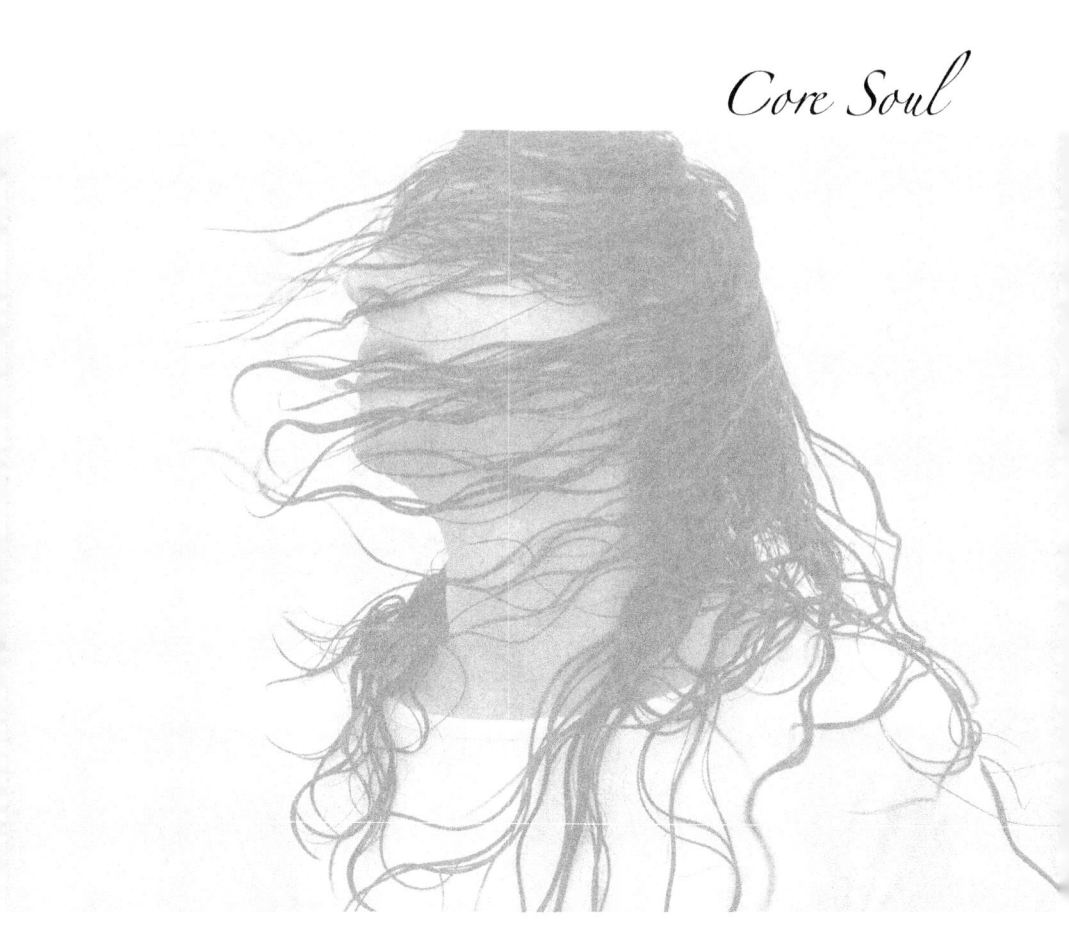

Core Soul

And those who were seen dancing were thought to be insane by those who could not hear the music.

– Friedrich Nietzsche

The Meaning of the Soul

> My brain is only a receiver. In the Universe there is a core from which we obtain knowledge, strength and inspiration. I have not penetrated into the secrets of this core, but I know it exists.
>
> —Nikola Tesla

So far, the journey of core healing has taken us into the rich diversity of human existence. In Core Mind we explored the power of the conditioned belief systems that seemingly shape and control our lives. This was followed by Core Body, in which we embraced the body and the importance of its daily maintenance through a whole body detoxification program. We have also experienced how it feels to dance with a partner or to dance alone, to swirl with your eyes open or closed, to passionately surrender to the rhythm of the beating drums, or to gently follow the sweet sound of a single note like a swift ocean breeze. We have covered a lot of material so far, and I congratulate all of you who are still willing to go another step further regarding your core healing. Again, this book is not meant to be a step-by-step manual on how to free yourself from your mental, emotional, or physical illness, but to provide you with an overall understanding what it takes to truly embrace lasting, effective, and transformative healing in today's world.

Core Soul

As we enter Core Soul, you will dance through a magic world of imagination that enables you to see the entire spectrum of your personality, which longs to be healed and reunited with your soul again. Here, you will dance with your partner within, a dance that will ultimately become your eternal dance throughout your life.

Let's start by imagining you are about to return to your beloved home after having traveled for a very long time. You might have been abroad and lived among different cultures or experienced a very difficult time away from your loved ones due to political circumstances like war or living in exile. Now, here you are... about to embrace your loved ones once again and enter the familiar environment you once called home. Your heart, your spirit, and your entire being is bursting with joy and excitement, rejoicing in this very moment of contentment and happiness. You, your mind, body, and soul have come home, and you are dancing with yourself again.

In June 2007, I had a dream that planted the seed for this book and served as my general vision and understanding of transformative and effective treatments. Some nights are like no others, and this night was one of those times when I recognized that a meaningful and profound transmission had been communicated to me. Was my highest intelligence speaking to me... or had I heard the voice of my soul, emerging from its depth and entering into my consciousness while I was asleep? I don't have a clear answer to this question, yet I am keenly aware of the importance of the message, trusting its validity and source of origin. In my dream I heard, "Angelika, true healing has to go beyond the actual cause of each case history."

"What do you mean by that?" I asked the seemingly higher presence.

"It means you have to go beyond the actual symptom and the cause, possibly far beyond, to the very point where the individual patient hasn't yet embraced his or her physical form. To that very point where the human in need was still a sphere, or a ball of light, an energy

Core Soul

force carrying a nucleus, the very soul and core of him or herself. Going back in time, in this center of light-energy an explosive division occurred, which ultimately became the separation of the soul from source itself. You will have to go back to the point of division, to this very core of deep loss and deviation from the self. This is true healing! This will be the future medicine."

As I pondered this incredible information, I wondered if this "center, or nucleus, of light-energy" represented the birthing pool of our creative intelligence, which after the split ultimately got separated from the soul and the whole. I didn't know the answer then and still don't, but I never forgot this unusual message. It was only recently, as I undertook the writing of this book, that I began to fully understand and appreciate its true significance.

In *Core Soul* I start by separating the subject of the soul into different parts before bringing bring them back together again. Know that what may initially seem like an unresolvable puzzle will eventually emerge as a completely new transformative experience.

ॐ

To talk about the soul is really difficult. Each attempt to describe one aspect of this multifaceted concept only highlights a number of others, so that we never quite manage to even skim the surface of what it means. Some talk about "having a soul"; others view the soul as a deeper core inside themselves. Either way, both concepts consider the soul or some aspect thereof as the source of divinity itself or a connection with it.

My favorite Irish author John O'Donohue speaks eloquently about the soul in this way: "Your soul knows the geography of your destiny. Your soul alone has the map of your future; therefore you can trust this indirect, oblique side of yourself. If you do, it will take you where you need to go, but more important it will teach you a kindness of rhythm in your journey."

My research and understanding of the nature of having or being a soul, started with a patient of mine.

Over the last three years a woman in her early 50s had struggled with her divorce and displayed strong emotional outbursts and a paradoxical behavior relative to her thinking and emotional patterns. As she described it, one day she felt she could handle it all and the next, provoked, she'd turn into someone altogether unrecognizable, someone engulfed by unbearable grief and rage. This patient was an intelligent and educated woman who very much understood her out-of-proportion reactions, but did not know how to change them. I had treated her with deep-acting homeopathy and she had attended regular therapy sessions with different psychotherapists, looked after herself by practicing yoga, and in general lived a healthy and nurturing life. As she hardly improved in all of her aspects, I began to think that I may have had prescribed the wrong homeopathic remedy or perhaps hadn't gone deep enough with my case analysis. Frustrated with the lack of progress, there were moments I almost gave up on her progress, as well as on my ability as a holistic health physician.

Over the years, any improvements the woman made were short-lived, only to be followed by endless falls back into her dark abyss. When I asked her to describe the experience of switching from a mature and collected person into a raging beast, she answered: "It is a force, it's something that just comes over me. I know it's wrong, but when it happens I can't do anything about it, it is much stronger than me. I think I have a very nasty depression, and that I've had it for a long time. My lows and highs, my destructive thoughts and behavior, my bad sleeping, my lack of seeing any sense in it all, and my lack of any hope for any meaningful future life are now a constant and daily part of me. I am stuck and have been for a long time. My thoughts are like a broken record in my head. I feel totally detached from reality. There's this terrible feeling inside of me that whatever I do or say makes not a jot of difference. My life is total crap. My mind is overactive and critical. I go over and over the same stuff—what he [husband] did and said—and I am haunted by everything."

I then remembered another patient who had been plagued with a delusional sexual perversion describing a similar experience. He also mentioned an inexplicable force, "a rush of energy that just came over him," during which he felt so helpless that he complied with whatever this force "wanted him to do."

Core Soul

The medical literature may have defined these strong emotional and mental states in diagnostic terms like bipolar disorder or manic depression or schizophrenia. And perhaps an orthodox medical practitioner would have been content to label such behavior as one of these diseases to justify a prescribed medication.

Well, I wasn't content to do so. I wanted to know and understand what was really happening here. Were these patients talking about an uncontrollable addiction or mental obsession? I needed to get to the bottom of the nature of this powerful temptation that was ultimately making them lose their authentic power, as it is my belief that unless we start to understand the dynamic that underlies the phenomenon of addiction, we will never be able to release it.

Beneath every addiction is the perception that the use of the drug or the drink or the pill offers us a chance to become more powerful and mightier. That somehow we will be, at least momentarily, connected with a power greater than ourselves. Yet our acting out through addiction is simply a way to exert the control we feel we lack over the people and situations in our external world. Beneath every addiction lies this unresolved issue of the love of power. My female patient undoubtedly felt powerful as long as she claimed and identified with her state of mental and emotional frenzy. In that moment when she allowed herself to yell and criticize her estranged husband, she really felt powerful, although far from living her truly authentic power. Acknowledging an addiction or accepting that you have an addiction is the first step in welcoming that part of you that behaves "out of control." Most of the time obsessional or addictive reactions are actually fueled by a deep-seated fear of losing that same control.

Today we know from studies that people who display out-of-control sexual behavior, for example, are really struggling with issues of power. Living in a place of self-inflicted addiction is not possible at the same time one is living in a place of true authentic power. The two cannot exist simultaneously.

Core Soul

The interesting fact regarding my female patient's emotional conflict revolved around her increasing desire to heal her mental and emotional addiction and increasing awareness of the cost of holding onto her apparently misguided power game. As her treatments unfolded, we both recognized that she had arrived at the door of decision: to either keep her addiction alive or begin walking a completely different path of life.

As a health practitioner, however, I was still relating to this case from an analytical perspective and trying to find an intellectual solution, either in the form of a natural, holistic prescription or counseling strategy. Until one day I found myself experiencing a similar mental and emotional trauma to the one that was enslaving my patient. Suddenly I knew what it felt like to feel trapped by my own constantly revolving mental negativity. And it was making my life a living hell.

❦

It all started after a terrible and very painful relationship breakup. Initially, I went through the familiar phases of shock, denial, grief, anger, resignation, and depression. Three years on, however, I still was in dire need of healing. At this point, even I recognized that my thought processes had become obsessive. I thought about my lost partner the minute I woke up until the minute I went to bed. My inner world revolved around countless imagined discussions with him in which I tried desperately to get my thoughts and feelings across in the hope of being understood. It had become a vicious, endless game of chasing my own tail. There were days I caught myself praying desperately for the final end of this mental tyranny.

I then realized that I was giving my mind and thoughts power and an identify of their own. They had become my oppressors and the embodiment of an entity of domination, an internally living beast that I had metamorphosed into a prostitute of my own creation. I was trapped inside myself: a prisoner of my own self-perpetuating thought processes and a slave of my own splintered personality. Some of you might recognize yourself here, as I imagine that during the course of our lives many of us have been there once or twice.

Core Soul

It was this experience that encouraged me to explore much more deeply the phenomenon of duality. It seemed to me that we have two simultaneous processes working: our thoughts and the level of consciousness we apply to those thoughts. The more I acknowledged that there might be two different worlds coexisting, but not always in agreement, in myself, the more I began to be able to step back and bear witness of my unfolding life. What was the spectrum of this turmoil? What was the true scope of my inner world?

Fascinated by the possibility of overcoming and transforming my mental tyranny, I dedicated an entire summer to reading and researching the nature of the soul, with only a brief interruption for my older son's wedding in the idyllic English countryside and a short trip to a beautiful crop circle to rest my head and body. Crop circles are formations created by the flattening of a crop such as wheat, barley, rye, maize, or rapeseed into geometrical shapes. Some believe as I do that crop circles transmit beneficial messages for humanity. I also took extra time to cleanse my body with the bountiful harvest of pears and apples from my garden and a nutritious, organic, raw food diet. Not a bad summer!

The more I studied the soul, relative to its religious, indigenous, and in-depth psychological aspects, I became distinctly aware of its inherent opacity. It seems the soul was impossible to pin down! Being brought up under the Roman Catholic influence, my idea of the soul mainly focused on something that was present after a human (or its shell) had passed away, a sort of etheric trail. Yet, as I continued to look deeply into the nature of the soul, a completely new picture emerged that would profoundly change my relationship toward my conditioned belief system born of the past, and the relationship to my future. I had suddenly awakened to the possibility that I truly could influence my future path, my DNA, and my cellular behavior—and do it without necessarily always depending on holistic treatments.

I was, I am, and I became the remedy!

Core Soul

When we talk about the soul, many of us picture ourselves as having something that determines who we are at our depth, at the very core of ourselves, a place that is very close to our inner truth. To have a soul or to lose a soul is a statement about authenticity, integrity, and virtue. When we are moved by a piece of music, watch an expressive dance performance, or listen to a deeply moving poetry reading, we talk about and experience this event as soul-full, as something real, uncluttered, pure, or untouchable. When we speak of soul music, we all know and feel the meaning underlying its expression. It is music that speaks from the heart and the very core of its creator, who is unafraid to expose his or her feelings about life itself. To betray or hurt a soul certainly has long-term, deep repercussions. We speak of how a soul "has moved on" once its human shell has died, seemingly detaching itself from its host and floating into other realms in order to continue the course of its "life." We also address the meaning of the soul when we start questioning our purpose in life or our very existence on Earth.

In fact, due to the current inner and external paradigm shifts, many people have started asking themselves questions like: Who am I? What is my purpose of my life? What is my true assignment if it is more than an obligation to a job or external expectations that do not serve me anymore?

Each of us is increasingly contemplating how this New World will unfold and how our individual lives will be affected by this global change in process. Right now, most of us are interested in initiating contact with this emerging force called change that we can see in our global political uproars, the general intolerance of outlived patterns of ignorance, and the lies reflected in the daily news and our individual stories. We all are striving for more authenticity, trying to live a more humane life. Some of us might view this as the hardest time to live, but others as the greatest privilege to be alive and fortunate enough to see the transformation.

There is no other time like now. We are indeed in a time of deep change! I believe you and the world and I are searching for fulfillment and a deeper purpose. And that perhaps the search itself will ultimately become the real purpose of life. I do know that the deepest longing of the human soul is to be seen and that now is the time to make that happen.

Core Soul

Through my studies, I learned that we are indeed born with a soul, and that the new paradigm encourages us to become active participants in living a soulful and soul-full life.

Our souls are also yearning for a deeper meaning and purpose, an identity that not only expresses an authentic relationship to us and to life, but to a deliberate, sustainable quality of life. In my community, many of my friends and I are downsizing our material possessions, giving away assets we don't need anymore, and organizing countless yard sales to de-clutter our already abundant lives. We all feel the need to create an externally clean and unburdened space in order to better sense and navigate our evolutionary journeys toward a direction that takes us far into the depth of ourselves. Our souls are ready to heal!

The journey of healing the soul is demanding and not an easy path. Why? As you are asked to exercise a life with mindfulness, you are also asked to apply your awareness to each and every aspect of your life. To live a soulful life, you will have to give up your addictive thought processes and actions.

The Roman emperor Marcus Aurelius once stated: "The soul becomes dyed with the color of its thoughts," meaning that your responsibility today is to see and witness the hue as well as the context of your mental circus. This is the very first step toward any transformation.

In the words of Alan Watts, British philosopher, writer, and speaker: "The only way to make sense of out of change is to plunge into it, move with it and join the dance." This is the reason I believe in your dance. I believe we are hardwired to transform.

The fundamental belief that the soul and body are separate from each other governs overall general opinion on this subject to this day. Yet, numerous cultures have shared their wisdom with us in support of the knowledge that humans are made of both body and soul together. In fact, certain tribal cultures have located the soul to a particular organ within the body, like the heart or liver, or to the entire bloodstream. Other tribes choose the breath as the expression of the soul, what the Greeks referred to as the psyche, or spirit. The Romans believed that the soul left the dying person with his last breath to continue its journey outside the bounds of physical form.

Core Soul

The idea that the soul is separate from the body was initially imprinted by the ancient Greeks and then later adopted and carved in stone by the universal Christian movement. In Christianity, the meaning of the soul became a fundamental principle of immortality as portrayed through one's ongoing endeavor to repent one's sins, as only through repentance can the soul ascend to an imaginary "heaven." Other traditional cultures claim we have more than one soul, confusing this mental construct even more. Overall, however, there remains a general consensus that at some point the soul detaches itself from the body, either through death or psychological trauma.

Living in a high-desert mountain community, my spiritual path, and to some extent my expression of life, has been influenced by its Native American culture. The land that embraces my home and clinic once belonged to the Tewa and Apache Indians with their deep-rooted Earthbound relationship to Nature. The Native American teachings speak of a person suffering from illness or emotional trauma by referring to him as a "lost soul" unable to find his way back home. Here, it is the role of the shamanic healer to support the individual's journey of retrieving the soul that has wandered off. Once the lost soul is found and has returned to its human host for reattachment, a smooth and complete recovery can begin on the mental, emotional, and/or physical levels.

I have witnessed this phenomenon in both children and adults who have been exposed to severe sexual abuse, physical or emotional violence, over-prescribed drugs therapies, and excessive recreational substance use. In these instances, the soul chooses to detach itself from the body as a means of survival. Looking into the eyes of a sexually abused girl or boy, particularly in the case of young children, you can easily recognize the soulless eyes embedded in a soulless body. Such children are barely surviving their unfolding futures.

Today, it is not only afflicted children and adults who are showing signs of a separated soul or of having lost their way. However, the vast majority of humanity may not even recognize its strong yearning for integration, for a merging with their unique and awaiting soul. When humanity does realize this need and desire, each personal connection will ultimately begin to catalyze humanity's connection with the larger soul of the whole world.

Core Soul

Our beliefs about the soul have undergone many shifts through the years. At some point we stopped viewing the soul as an integrated element of the body and began seeing it as separate from the body. We labeled the bodily element "mortal" and the soul element "immortal." In time, Christianity adopted this idea of a divided soul and body, laying the foundation for a deeply imprinted, yet disconnected cellular relationship toward the body and toward life itself. Unfortunately, widespread religion today has forgotten that heaven is not a place, but a daily practice in state of mind.

The idea that the soul is somehow in conflict with the body is attributed to Orpheus, a figure in Greek mythology who descended into Hades, the underworld abode of the souls of the dead, to retrieve his wife. Orpheus teaches us that the soul is able to detach itself from the body and exist totally independently as an out-of-body state. This ideology had a profound influence on Pythagoras, Greek philosopher and mathematician and my favorite healer and shaman. In my view, Pythagoras is the key innovator of homeopathy and general alternative medicine. Pythagoras believed that animals share the privilege of having a soul with us. Plato's pupil Aristotle, although not his follower, changed our viewpoint again, stating that the soul was another form of the body. Aristotle strongly advocated that the soul was inseparable from the body and therefore of a mortal nature: He stated: "It is absurd as to say that the art of carpentry could embody itself in flutes. Each art must use its tools, each soul its body."

To Aristotle, the soul radiated the essential "whatness," or its body's character, and was the cause for, or source of, the living body. In order to connect with the soul, he said we need our senses and imagination, not our thinking processes; that we touch and express the soul through our senses. Aristotle tells us: "Since nothing except what is alive can be fed, what is fed is the besouled body and just because it has soul in it. Hence food is essentially related to what has soul in it."

The search to understand the concept of the soul has continued from the 15th century to today. It is an ongoing dance! Numerous attempts were made to describe and formalize the concept of the soul far into the 19th century, particularly by Sigmund Freud, father of psychoanalysis, and C. G. Jung, psychologist and psychiatrist, who presented the character of the soul not as a means of reason but by its approach through the imagination. This idea represented a totally new way of thinking and profoundly changed our relationship to our body and soul once again.

After weeks exploring all manner of the written word about the soul, it became clear to me that the whole dialogue in defining the soul, stretching over hundreds of years, was ultimately focused on the primal conflict of personal power versus authentic power. People who choose to act from the realm of lower frequencies, or their shadow sides, have the objective to conquer and win, whatever it takes, whatever the cost. The still deeply embedded theory of the survival of the fittest comes to the forefront in this way.

It appears that an almost schizophrenic mental war is going on, one that deeply reflects a humanly intrinsic and ego-driven mechanism. Compelled by the ego's resistance of the soul, our personalities become distorted. This pervading sense of distortion and contention then consistently continues to govern our daily behaviors. The more I delved into my own inner war of this kind, the more it led me to think about the global agony of so many individual scarred souls and a scarred world that manifests its lack of oneness through endless wars and self-inflicted destructiveness. Sadly, such inflated, determined battles only result in the loss of individual and community power. Is it not a common sentiment that we feel drained, leached of our personal power—that it seems we have given it away?

With each choice you make, you either align yourself with the energy of your soul or with your distorted personality, your ego. The ruthless temptations of our thought processes desire nothing more than to be seen and hailed as victorious rulers of their conquered territory. As soon as you give in to your addictive behaviors and conditioned, negative thought processes, you freely give yourself the permission to be irresponsible. But these niggling temptations—and addictions—are not only resisting your attempts to merge with your soul, but are the very parts of you in most need of healing. Beneath every addictive thought process and behavior reins the king or queen in the relentless pursuit of power. Underlying every crisis, particularly emotional crisis, sits the issue of power.

The very reason my female patient couldn't break through her addictive emotional patterns was that she was really unwilling to let go off her possessive position of power and dominance. It is only by taking the journey to understand the dynamics of our personality and the purpose of our soul that we can begin to see the absurdity of this life-long inner battle. Embracing true freedom requires breaking through your defenses and beyond to consciously experience the nature of your darker aspects and accept a different kind of power—the power to change them. The purpose of your life is to emancipate yourself from your mental slavery.

My deeper understanding led me to welcome a different kind of power that embraces and loves life in all its forms, a power free of judgment and allows meaningfulness in all the Earth provides. As soon as we choose to deviate from our personal power games, we can enter the realm of authentic power, whose roots are planted in the deepest source of our being. Authentic power can't be bought, sold, or dressed in corporate attire. Authentic power emerges from a place of truth and integrity.

We are all encouraged to engage in this universal consciousness shift, from a species pursuing external power into one that integrates and becomes authentically empowered. Some authors describe this metamorphosis as shifting from living in our current five-sensory human state to living in a multi-sensory state. From the perception of a limited sensory human, life is based on what we see, what we are dealing with, a rational world based on reasoning that does not generally include the so-called "imaginary" or spirit world. In this realm of reason, intentions have no effect and the world is addressed based on a perspective of sheer mental and emotional practicality.

For the awakened being using multiple senses, daily life is filled with numerous learning experiences. Internally and externally encountered situations as well as people serve as mirrors of experience to support the individual's evolutionary growth. In this New World, every intention has an effect. Our decisions, yours and mine, affect us and the lives of everyone and everything else in this realm. They reach far beyond this physical world.

In this New World, your decisions and actions determine your evolution. There is no need to blame the external world for, nor feed it with, your negative or conditioned projections. In this New World, you are the author of your story. You might think that sounds too new age or like a rose-colored vision, but consider the fact of physics. You might be just a drop in this vast ocean we call life, but imagine the ripple one drop can cause! I recently read this apt American proverb: "It all boils down to your perception and how you want to relate to your life, as the only difference between stumbling blocks and stepping stones is the way in which we use them."

Soul can't be identified by any literal approach or attempts to describe it in religious or philosophical terms.

Patrick Harpur in *The Complete Guide to the Soul* writes: "The soul's separateness from the body is a metaphor for its reluctance to be defined and pinned down in a single image. As the very thing, which sees through everything else, soul is not itself anything. It takes on the coloration of whatever image is currently embodying it. The very word soul is an image for itself, which itself is empty, like the Tao, drawing its substance from whatever forms it assumes. Soul cannot be known objectively, only subjectively through reflections and insights. We cannot step outside soul to study her. She is a way of looking at all disciplines and thus hidden within every field of inquiry."

☙

We are all soul, and our body radiates its soulful embodiment. We may all be individual souls, yet we simultaneously embody a unified world soul at the same time, a state C. G. Jung describes as the "collective unconscious." None is excluded nor preferred here, as we are all sitting and rowing in the same boat called life. Soul, not body alone, has always been and always will be the source of life. This planet and realms beyond are penetrated by and imbued by its vibration.

Until now, we may have never truly contemplated the possibility of being and living as autonomous and free soul-beings or what it would be like to be fully conscious of our limited mental core belief systems while being fully engaged in the process of healing. Such an engagement would certainly result in a very different outer world. There is a big difference between relating to the world without awareness and actively and consciously participating in it.

When you feel your soul, when you live through your soul, you turn an ordinary event into an experience that includes your senses and feelings. This act infuses each moment with its depth, its quality, its flavor, and character. I think of this frequency as the frequency of love. Though often indescribable or intangible, the feeling of love can be fully lived and expressed through every cell of our being. It is by feeling this vibration that you come to experience the energy of the soul.

Your soul is not a passive or a theoretical entity occupying an anatomical part of your body; it is a life-changing and purposeful force at the very core of your being. You cannot get to know your soul through the objective path of mental and theoretical analysis; it can only be met through reflection, insight, and imagination. Think about this! When we talk about the soul, we are exploring what it says about itself through you! The soul is not separate from you, but reflects you! We therefore cannot step outside the soul to get to know it. Only by consciously surrendering to it can we see the inner priestess within consistently healing us to wholeness.

Isn't it time for us to stop trying to win this doomed battle over the "nature" of the soul and instead learn how to become one with it and live from that boundless and luminous place? To get to know your soul takes courage, perseverance, and determination in the face of adversity while you become your own humble witness to your inner shadows. To become a soulful being, you have to commit yourself to the willingness to distill, cleanse, and purge yourself each and every day from your mental, emotional, and physical toxicity. If you want to change your life and your physical illness, it takes every bit of your soul to make that change.

To get to know and commune with your soul, the first step is to recognize that you have a soul. Ask yourself: What does my soul look like; what is its nature? Who is my soul? What is the voice of my soul? What is its language? How does my soul influence my life? What is my belief about the soul? Do I see it as an integrated part of myself or do I only relate to it as something that will leave my body after my death?

If we accept the concept of the soul as something that leaves upon death, this might also imply that we accept the current immature civilization that manipulates our reality. Do we fail to see how it distorts and blinds us with tantalizing carrots that dangle right in front of our eyes and lead us astray, rather than inward toward our true soul and the soul of this world? Once you recognize the energy of your soul, its value and essential purpose will begin the process of merging with the life of your distorted personality, or small self. At this point, you become less and less interested in feeding this internal entertainment of who will win the ongoing battle and more interested in witnessing the embodiment of your personality into a frequency of service to the life of your soul. At this point the ego that was only interested in the self-centered desire for victory will align willingly with the soul's vast experiences and leave behind the addictive striving and obsession for personal power. It is then that authentic power can stream into and color your life. Then, all limitations cease to exist!

As I continued pondering how to truly help my female patient, I understood that if she were to completely heal her mental and emotional suffering through a breakthrough, she would have to be willing to walk the path to find and accept her soul. In essence, she would have to participate in her soul's awakening. Since the natural remedies and treatments appeared to have come to a momentary halt in their effectiveness, we would have to embark on the next part of our uncharted territory, the place within, the journey of the soul.

In *Spontaneous Evolution* Bruce H. Lipton and Steve Bhaerman encourage us in this way: "Those willing to face the music and dance together will be the ones who will help transform the threatening crises we face into awesome opportunities. Even though Nature is nudging us toward this exciting possibility it cannot happen without our participation. We are conscious co-creators in the evolution of life. We have free will. And we have choices. Consequently our success is based on our choices, which are, in turn, totally dependent on our awareness."

Core Soul

My female patient had described herself as going insane and questioning the existence of her life, just as I once had done. Surely, the answer was to be found in making the choice to become sane!

☙

Our journey has taken us through the mind, the body, and now the soul. We have entered an exciting and literally mind-blowing experience, which will slowly add the final pieces to your complete core healing. Are you still ready to dance?

Imagine you are attending a public dance or a party. Your eyes can't help noticing the attractive young woman or the gorgeous young man across the other side of the room. In your mind, you already envision yourself talking, laughing, or perhaps dancing with your dream-woman or dream-man, yet shyness is holding you back from making your mental images come true. I hereby invite you to summon all your courage and walk up to your other half, to your dream's coming alive. Gently take his or her hand as you walk to the dance floor, knowing that this step is full of opportunity and that you have just fulfilled your dream, right here, right now.

To change, a person must face the dragon of his appetites with another dragon, the life-energy of the soul.

—Rumi

The Authentic Dance beyond Yourself

> There is no coming to consciousness without pain. People will do anything, no matter how absurd, in order to avoid facing their own soul. One does not become enlightened by imagining figures of light, but by making the darkness conscious.
>
> —Carl Gustav Jung

How does it feel to dance with your Self? You have learned how to dance with an external partner, to dance alone, and now you are learning to dance with your internal partner, the most precious, the most beautiful, the most authentic lover you will ever embrace and cherish. Start describing your dance partner. How does he or she look? How is he/she dressed? What color is his/her hair? Tell him/her how beautiful he/she looks today. Tell him/her that you have waited for him/her and this dance for a very long time. Tell him/her that there is no other, that he/she is the very one. The search to find your lifelong soul mate is finally over as you softly fall into your inner peace. In this state of bliss, your heart and body tremble with such blazing vibrancy that any moment you could burst and flow over with love. Here you are; you have arrived at the point where you can allow yourself to dance with your body and soul and beyond.

For this dance, choose a very special place, a place that is very dear to your heart. You take only your closest loved ones and friends there, as this sacred place resonates with your energy field; it is your external and internal sanctuary. It may be your favorite spot on the river, an overlook at a spectacular valley, a meadow behind your house, or your living room, designed with your sense of beauty and with your expression of love.

In order to be authentic, to be real, to be yourself, hold nothing back and dare to go beyond yourself to a place you have never gone before. A place where you can't hold yourself together anymore, a place where you willingly want to lose control, as you are now fueled with your deepest yearning to dance with your soul. You are your soul and your soul is you.

In the previous chapter I talked about the meaning of "soul" based on many different concepts that have unfolded through the ages. Today, we have arrived at a completely new paradigm in our relationship to the soul and to the body. Here, ancient scriptures and ideologies must be put aside in order to claim and integrate a newfound communication within. This includes setting a firm commitment to stop feeding our mental and emotional projections to the outside world.

How would your life look if you once and for all stopped blaming and criticizing your spouse, your boss, your children, your mother-in-law, or your environment? True commitment is not based on your personal wishes or desires, but is unconditional in nature. True commitment . . . just is. But our conditioned belief systems create vacillating attitudes of self-doubts, ambivalence, worry, anxiety, and—most significantly—fear. To learn to dance with your soul you will need to set a different mental and emotional stage where you alone represent the world in which you live and the world with which you engage. It is time to stop blaming external situation for your internal misery.

This doesn't mean you are not allowed to express your feelings when somebody has done you wrong or has hurt you. On the contrary, I would encourage you to express your feelings and clearly present your boundaries, trying not to condemn the soul of the perpetrator, but only his or her actions. Once we learn to get in touch with and listen to the silence within, knowing that everything in life has a purpose, then there are no mistakes, there are no coincidences, and everything is offered to us as a learning experience. That which now appears to threaten your comfort and stability has the capacity to become the reason why the future is bright. That's it! The drama stops right there and then! Your task in life is not to seek your happiness through your loved ones, your profession, or your external world, but to explore and be willing to break through the personal barriers that are keeping you from living a liberated and healthy life.

Our conditioned ingrained belief systems, thoughts, and actions are not separate aspects of the soul, but more like offshoots of it. These splintered aspects in dire need of healing need to interact with the physical realm so that each part of the distorted self can become whole again. The personality looks like a multifaceted intricately woven tapestry with countless multicolored threads, each one representing our conditioned thought patterns and perceptions about life. Yet, in this stunning masterpiece of a tapestry, we also find many other threads already radiating their completeness. We might call this tapestry our "awakened personality." The totality of this unique tapestry, with all its different parts, can be seen as the soul. If we begin to perceive uncomfortable thoughts and emotions triggered by unconsciously chosen mirrored life experiences as the impetus to awaken our true nature, we are more likely to accept them as aspects of the soul and not separate entities of our existence. In this context, our dysfunctional past, struggles, and pain all serve as nurturing fertilizer for personal transformation.

The moment the ancient cultures deviated and separated themselves from their cores, which manifested as personality versus soul, a deep misunderstanding emerged that would influence us for centuries. But there is no separation; there never was!

When Adam chose to eat the apple in the Garden of Eden he was infused by his ego's desire and temptations, consciously choosing to give his splintered personality more power than his soul. With this act, he gave his energy and power away. Yet his temptation was not a separate part of his soul, but a denser, more tangible form, teaching him to work with these frequencies with mindfulness and awareness instead of from the outlook of an ego fueled with insatiable addictions.

Core Soul

When we are universally separate from the whole, either through personality conditioning, chemicals, or pharmaceutical drugs (created by extracted selected substances rather than from the totality of the whole healing plant), and a disassociated life, we are doomed to live out our self-inflicted daily crises. The whole is always greater than the sum of its parts. This split from the whole has consequences and taints our entire life. Remember that such seemingly tragic moments are actually directly born from parts of the soul that it has chosen to heal in this lifetime. Can you see and understand the purpose of your soul now?

The soul, even without specific form, lives in the here and now, and continues to express its wholeness through its entirety. Therefore, the distorted personality emerges as a natural energy, or force, from the soul. It is not, nor has it ever been separate from its very core. Your soul has consciously chosen all its aspects in order to live and function in a healthier and more sustainable future. Sound, color, and matter are made of the same energetic components as the soul. The only difference is in density and consistency, depending on the chosen realm of manifestation. The same principle applies to your personality, which is unable to function independently of your soul because it is an aspect of your soul.

Gary Zukav, in *The Seat of the Soul*, offers this poignant comment: "The dynamic of the soul and personality is the same dynamic as energy converted into matter. The system is identical. Your body is your matter. Your personality is the energy of your soul converted into matter. If it is unaware, it is the splinteredness that is transmitted. If it is aware, it begins to become whole."

જી

Today, our planetary conflicts are directly and proportionally related to the extent and severity of humanity's separation from its soul, as are our personal conflicts directly related to our ability or inability to live a conscious life through the soul. It is very clear that our personal evolution directly affects the evolution of humanity and vice versa. When a person lives and expresses himself in a balanced and healthy way, there is no real line between the personality and the soul. When we recognize ourselves in everything we will be inspired to exercise true equality (and equanimity) and dismantle the ongoing wars into constructive and fruitful dialogues.

Such balance involves seeking the meeting point of our self-created polarities, the place where two different realms seem to operate at the same time, in order to achieve our one purpose: unification. Equanimity can be cultivated when we stop judging and/or identifying ourselves with whatever happens to us. To become an active participant in the creation of this New World, we are encouraged to live from the center of ourselves, to dance in the middle of our personal dance floor rather than squirm around its edges trying to manipulate life, whose goal for us is to be spontaneous, wild, and free.

Just as two magnets will never come together at their similar poles, opposites, or polarities and will never unite, we must learn to integrate both valuable poles, negative and positive, to design a functional and authentic world.

❧

With this newfound knowledge, my life was bound to change. It had to. Once you know that there is no separation between the self's mental tyranny, based on fear, criticism, anger/rage, and judgment—all aspects about which one feels guilty and ashamed of and the luminous soul—you cannot go back. At this point I began experimenting with a daily exercise, one that I still use whenever I feel myself drifting back into my mental craziness. I imagine I am a bird, an eagle, soundlessly gliding over my unhealed personality and my soul at the same time. As the eagle is the bird that flies higher than any other bird the sky, it therefore flies closest to the sun. In my opinion, this means it must have the best view for taking in the entire spectrum of life around it.

I started with my bruised personality, which was now ready to change. In my mind, I circled over and over the person called Angelika, who I recognized as feeling angry and betrayed. I saw her stomping on the floor like the mistreated and misunderstood child as she was, kicking and screaming loud accusations. There I was, arguing and defending myself to my imaginary ex-partner, trying to win this verbal air-battle. And the more I realized the chance of winning was slim, the more my mind got even more fired up in its attempt to come up with even better reasons, negotiations and arguments. It was like being in my own courtroom, trying to defend myself from my perpetrator and being the criminal at the same time.

Seeing myself from this perspective was a sad and humorous experience at the same time. I was witnessing Angelika literally chasing her own tail of mental and emotional tyranny, believing she was reaching her goal of victory. But from this perspective, Angelika's limited and self-imposed life had begun looking rather small. I was stunned to see that this rather self-limited experience, called Angelika's life, was the declaration of my reality, of my world. The truth was that all Angelika was doing was feeding off her emotional fire, reigniting the flames with self-perpetuating thought patterns in order to keep her false identity alive. I was that hamster running around in circles on its little plastic wheel, believing it was actually covering enormous time and distance.

What was I doing? Who was this person called "me," living this strange reality show, expecting that everyone around me liked it or even wanted to sign up to play a part in it?

While I was witnessing, allowing myself to be an objective observer, it occurred to me that I was still applying judgment and criticism according to my habits and conditioning. Only this time I was judging my distorted personality like a frustrated parent whose son or daughter hasn't fulfilled his dream or the miserable boss who expects more from his employee. When we judge, we create negative cause and effect patterns called karma. Judgment belongs to the personality, not to the soul.

Which brings me to the theme of expectation and how expectations have ramifications.

❧

Why do we constantly not only expect and demand the highest standards from ourselves but also project these ideals onto the outside world? "He didn't finish the task the way I wanted him to do!" "She wasn't up to scratch!" "He doesn't have the courage!" "She is unfit to be a mother!" He...she...it's an endless circus of awaited and failed expectations. What if our lives weren't subjected to expectations anymore? We could still strive for excellence and embrace the masterpiece we already are, but perhaps be more inclined to drop our fixed ideas about how the world should revolve around us. How about: "Don't expect anything"? Expectations are an attempt to control the future, a clear setup for likely failure when the imagined goal isn't met. Let's stay open-minded, fluid, and flexible to whatever life brings us and start our days with: "Hello new day, surprise me today...let's see what you've got for me!" A life based on non-judgment and non-attachment allows us to see freely without bringing negativity to the dance.

As soon as I welcomed the subtlety of this aspect of myself, something quite beautiful emerged. While watching my personal blockbuster in front of me, I deeply connected with a place within me that can only be described as pure compassion. At this moment, my heart literally overflowed with love and sweetness for this aspect of mine that was desperately trying to make a life based on purpose and values. Perhaps for the very first time, I felt forgiveness for her and for me and for all her past actions, which had resulted in the bitter aftertaste of her life.

In this very moment, I stepped into my other polarity called the soul; an infinite space filled with nothing tangible, yet everything I could ever have imagined. In this very moment, I chose to step out of my so-called petty and self-destructive world into a spacious boundlessness of just being. In this moment, everything was in its perfect place, at the perfect time, in its perfect condition without the need to justify, rectify, or demonstrate my point of view.

Thinking back to my female patient who was struggling so desperately with her uncontrollable outbursts, I now could clearly understand her dilemma. Her resistance to letting go of her identified personality had become her true illness and dis-ease. It was like sand slipping through her fingers. Already her hands displayed a chronic eczema with unbearable itchiness aggravated by her emotional instability and exposure to Nature's elements, like washing her hands with water. I understood so compassionately her feeling that if she were willing to let go of her negative and self-destructive energy field she might be lost in a void with nothing to hold onto anymore, not even her false identity.

This discussion brings us to the most human, primal core element of all: fear. Life is unable to progress in the midst of fear. Fear stops you in your tracks and warps you. Fear is the trap, intentionally placed to catch you and keep you inside your distorted personality.

*

The journey in becoming whole demands the journey of coming home to the soul. To fully embody the soul, the ego also must experience and feel the repercussions of its actions. The distorted parts of the personality serve as triggers to initially unbalance the soul as it asks to be healed and then, over time, pave the path to complete healing. Whether the soul is engaged in its healing path depends on the awareness of its awakened personality, or the capacity of the personality to go beyond itself. Each and every experience provides us with another opportunity to respond from the place of the soul or from the unhealed personality. The law of cause and effect then becomes the gift to one's divinity. This journey of giving birth to true authentic Self is called choice. The authentic Self is the soul made visible.

As we become conscious of every part of our self, our intentions and choices will manifest. Our true essential Self, once we know who we are, has the freedom to change, to let go of everything that is not essential to its well-being. Then the moments of doubt and indecision become fleeting moments of the past. As soon as we step away from our identification with the distorted self, we become responsible beings with the ability to make responsible choices for the world and ourselves.

Not to choose between the two, or to choose to live a life as a victim, is like living life as a Ping Pong ball in a self-created schizophrenic world where we give the soul away and allow ourselves to be drained of our authentic power. As soon as we become aware of the life and purpose of the personality, initially to heal and consequently to merge back into its source of origin, the soul, future choices begin to speak of a higher quality and depth. Each decision, from then on, determines the direction and place of perception from which we want to live.

A responsible choice takes into account the consequences of each action, fueled either by the mind or heart. From this perspective, we rarely feel overwhelmed or unprepared when life presents us with unexpected scenarios as we can handle such challenging event with a more composed maturity. Why not? Each and every one of us has written our individual script in the first place. Remember, there is no blame, there are no projections, only a courageous attitude in accepting the entire spectrum of initial choices. You are free to choose, but you are not free from the consequences of your choices.

Whenever you see yourself making a decision, ask yourself: *Is this particular project healthy for me? Does it serve my well-being and does it serve the world? Is this situation life affirming or is it life depleting?* What really matters is not so much what we do as how we do it. Are we acting consciously or are we reacting to some trigger? As we learn and train ourselves to live and respond from the soul, we simultaneously enter the realm of conscious transformation. Authentic power is an expression of living a soulful life, free of poking temptations and addictions, yet fully integrated and acknowledged within the living being. On the other hand, the distorted personality is only interested in itself, without concern for the well-being of its host, the soul, and the world. Its satisfaction is based on filling its self-orientated, insatiable form, its true gluttony. As long as we identify with its life and content, we give our power away, and continue to experience ourselves as victims, the one who is hard done by. Our responses to life experiences determine our future, not the actual experiences themselves.

The body primarily sickens or weakens depending on its host's choice to respond to life with a constricted energy or to adapt to the surrounding environment in more of a free-flowing way. As soon as we become the witness of our splintered personality, conscious of its ongoing struggle with itself, and evoke compassion and forgiveness for every part of our being, we can deviate from the need to create karmic lessons in order to awaken.

Core Soul

After some time training myself to choose a life based on responsible choices, I heard myself saying: "My karma is over!" I knew I no longer had to create these horrible and tortured situations in order to evolve. I was free! I thought this statement rather bold at first. After all, who was I to say such a thing? But I knew it was true. With that revelation also came the responsibility to use and apply my sharp discernment and eagle's eye and to leave my sweet naiveté behind. From now on, each and every choice had to be met with mindfulness and clarity. In this way, I didn't ignore my temptations, nor did I suppress or judge them; I simply chose not to act on them for the sake of my well-being and the sake of being an active part in creating the New World. From now on, I would become the creator of each moment!

Epiphanies like these can be small or large steps to a major breakthrough. As you shift your attention to your soul, because it is not a conditioned aspect of you, you will feel an incredible sense of relief. In this way, you literally shatter your deep-seated, limited belief systems. In Rumi's words: "Dance until you shatter yourself."

ॐ

In the grand scheme of life, my petty story and mulling over of my past relationship started to seem much less important, losing its zest as I detached it from its desire of wanting to be special. In fact, it took on a very ordinary and neutral flavor. Choosing a life based on wisdom and awareness, we not only empower ourselves but also become our own masters by challenging our temptations and addictive behaviors once and for all. From that point of view, we are asked to accept that each and every one of us, none excluded, walks the same long road in merging our personality and soul. Creed, color, nation, level of intellect... all without differentiation. When you know this, you begin to feel compassion even for those for whom you may never previously have felt it. We all are evolving, here and now, at the same time!

Have you ever noticed how tired and exhausted you and your body feels after you give away your power or let yourself be drained by lower frequencies, either from people's emotional baggage or a negative energy field? We are beings created of light and consciousness.

Core Soul

The quality of your consciousness is in direct proportion to your experience of being aware. As you start evolving and your consciousness rises, your strength of presence and light increase as well. What you feel and express can be literally measured as a visible frequency. In the community of holistic medicine, we find devices like advanced biofeedback can translate these frequencies into a user-friendly language, which enables the practitioner then to integrate this information in the treatment plan. The Institute of HeartMath has provided invaluable scientific research in this field.

HeartMath's patented emWave technology represents a breakthrough in personal feedback and stress reduction technology. It has enlightened us to the fact that the electromagnetic field of the Earth has a direct relationship with the electromagnetic field of our heart, which is many times stronger than the electromagnetic field of our brain. Emotions are therefore waves of energy, which, according to their signature, display different kinds of frequencies. We feel uplifted by emotions of love, joy, or happiness and brought heavy and low by emotions of hate, anger, or jealousy. Our thought patterns can evoke an emotional frequency in us. But it is not our brain causing all this to happen—it is our thoughts that shape our neural networks. The quality of our perception to life and the expression of our thoughts affect the body's cellular behavior as well as the quality of human vibrations.

As we send out thoughts into the environment and universe, they gather energy and vibrate at a frequency identical to circumstances and people who reside on this same frequency. The higher the vibration the more positive-filled events or people appear. For lower-frequency beings and systems to survive, they must feed parasitically on higher-frequency systems or to evolve into higher consciousness. If the person's resistance to evolving is stronger than following the primal urge to grow, the person exposed to this lower vibration will feel the energetic impact of such encounters. No matter how aligned and centered we are the body will feel drained and tired. We say it all the time: "He drains my energy!" When we feel burned out or stressed, this initial symptomatology often stems from an accumulation of built-up, unresolved stagnated life experiences, manifested as energy currents, which either block us from living a joyful life or blow out like a volcanic eruption, manifesting as rage and nervous breakdowns.

In *Core Body*, I pointed out the significance of energy as a cellular fuel and the new scientific findings that most degenerating diseases, called mitochondrial diseases, with decreased cellular energy production are caused by either an insufficient transport system of nutrients or the inability of the cell to receive and exchange nutrients. You also might remember that each mitochondria, located inside the cell, produces ATP (Adenosine TriPhosphate), the existential fuel for the body to stay alive. When the molecule ATP is released, ready to be converted into usable energy, it splits into the combustible and explosive energy molecule called ADP (Adenosine DiPhosphate) and phosphorus. When ATP is reduced to ADP, tiny explosions of phosphorescent light are in play. These little light explosions reflect your radiance and reveal the fact that you are luminous light. The more we consciously cleanse the mind and body by elevating our awareness, nurturing ourselves with a light-filled nutrition, and detoxifying the physical body from accumulated and stagnant toxicity, the more we produce cellular fuel and light throughout our energetic bodies.

The quality of your relationship to your soul is directly related to the quality of your physical cellular makeup, despite genetic weaknesses. Your soul and your body work in partnership, and what a successful and efficient partnership it is! Your consciousness affects every cell in your body and every cell in your body affects your consciousness. When somebody speaks from his or her soul, you will feel it and you will not feel drained afterward. In fact, you will probably feel energized and inspired. If somebody uses you to offload his or her unresolved emotional drama, however, your energy level is likely to sink or contract, resulting in an unbalanced state of being. Of course, we could argue here and remind you about not protecting yourself from this sucking-out-of energy event. But consider that these situations often happen on a very subtle level; before we become aware that they're happening, the drainage process has already begun. And it can happen anywhere—in the subway, on the bus, at work, at home with your loved ones, speaking on the phone, or via planetary events of a political and environmental nature, like nuclear meltdowns, oceanic oil spills, and the intensified activity of solar flares.

Energy is everything as it is the essence of life. Each and every day, you have to make the decision how you use your given energy resources, either to apply them with mindful awareness or recklessly burn them up. Your choice to live from your splintered personality or from your soul determines the supply of your energy reserves, on the spiritual, mental, emotional, and physical levels.

During this historic time, our species is evolving from a denser frequency range into a much broader spectrum of higher frequencies. The person who is becoming aware of the presence of his soul radiates and emanates a purer and lighter frequency; it is a given fact. The rest of us feel more attracted or inspired by these people, as their light literally lifts us into higher vibrational places. To raise your core vibration, start living from a place of mindfulness, a place that is calmer, more peaceful, less cluttered and complicated. By understanding the law of vibration, you then can use all frequencies to your advantage.

When I speak about being and living an authentic life, I speak about going beyond our shadows and distorted personalities. Your dance can be seen as a meditation, a dance when you go beyond your thoughts, beyond your mind, and beyond your individuality, and allow yourself to merge with your soul. Then your dance isn't just a dance anymore; it has become your trance dance.

ॐ

The path to your soul is through your feelings. This is the only path that is able to connect you with your very core. To sense and live your soul you have to feel it; by using your feelings a magical door called liberation opens to a world of unlimited potentialities.

It is not uncommon for us to be asked to take on the soul journey through an intense circumstance or crisis in our lives, like the loss of a loved one, either human or animal, the shattering moment when we receive the diagnosis of a terminal disease, a spouse's unforeseen announcement of divorce, being fired from a job after years of dedication, or the loss of all material possessions due to an environmental disaster. These raw moments in life push us into a state of awareness beyond our personality as we are catapulted into a state of mental shock or emotional void. Yet these very painful experiences are precisely the triggers that say "Wake up!" Crushed and brought to our knees, we are reminded to evolve into more spiritual beings. In these shocking moments, we know we have lost control, whether internal or external, but usually a combination of both. But we also lose the false belief in our own feelings of what it means to be powerful in order to experience authentic power. However impossible it is to contemplate in advance, it is the nature of being human that we somehow find ourselves more open and able to access the true realm of empowerment when we are feeling such intense vulnerability.

In my practice I have found that this time of global and personal transformation is having a profound effect on my patients, who are showing signs of intensified emotional and physical symptoms. I have witnessed the separation and loss of so many relationships and marriages that one wonders if the human predicament of polarization can truly be healed in the time to come. As we slowly but surely shift from left brain thinking, the rational and more male-orientated faculty, to right brain-orientated thinking, the more intuitive, receptive, and feminine faculty, we also witness the stark polarization of these seemingly opposite forces that resist each other in a conflict against the inevitable changes.

The female principle embodies more of the internal, personal feelings in our experience, whereas the masculine principle focuses more on the outer world, the more rational world, by emphasizing the mental faculties. This polarization is being played out in each of our hearts, personalities, and souls, as it is between men and women. We are all influenced and asked to respond to this unstoppable force by recognizing and breaking down old paradigms of patriarchal authority figures and the old established order currently overwhelmed by left-brain thinking patterns.

Many men who come to my practice are feeling (perhaps for the first time) the collapse of their identified role as the one in power. As one patient told me: "I feel like I am losing my power!" When asked what he meant by "losing his power," he answered in a clear demonstration of how easy it is to fall under an illusion of what it really means to be powerful, "Nothing seems to work anymore. My family is falling apart. Having both a girlfriend and a wife.... Even my business doesn't give me the same spark anymore. I'm falling apart because I feel so powerless!" I couldn't help noticing that although this man was referring to his own personal situation he was also inadvertently describing the global collapse of our present patriarchal consciousness.

This is what I told him: "Until you surrender to the general female principle, Gaia, our Mother Earth, the receptive, the feeling aspect within yourself, as well as to your outer world, you will not embrace authentic power. Authentic power is not the same as "feeling powerful" in the way that you know it now. Reaching for your authentic power means bowing down to a greater force that is not necessarily only male in nature. When you surrender to your world within, a softer and more female-orientated journey will lead you to your evolved power. This is how you will learn to give up control over your distorted personality and discover a new kind of empowered living." My patient listened to my answer with a smile, and we both knew a seed had been planted.

As we enter the coming years with a newfound consciousness, we increasingly start asking ourselves: *Do I listen to my mind and rational reasoning or do I feel into my heart? Do I follow what is expected from me and therefore conform to social norms? Do I follow what is right and healthy for me or do I comply with the opinions of my peers without addressing myself regarding my needs? How can I become an individual fully able to express my creativity and at the same time participate as an active serving individual of this world?*

☙

As we slide through our own re-birthing process to live from a place deep inside where consciousness touches pure energy and where the core of primal energy touches consciousness, our planet Earth is also enduring her own long and painful labor pains.

Core Soul

During recent years we have been experiencing a shift in the Earth's magnetic polarization, a shift that takes place only once every 26,000 years and influences everything we experience. The magnetic shift of the Earth is central to an overall realignment of the universe as we know it. Even this "slight" movement ensures a new position that puts us in direct alignment to receive energy from as yet unknown parts of the universe at large. As new and vital information streams into the planet regarding its survival and our core well-being, change within us is imminent and inevitable.

As soon as we are willing to expand our perceptions we experience the changes that are afoot, most of the time to our betterment. In order to grow, however, we are encouraged to give up the struggle to remain the same by learning to embrace the situations that present themselves as vehicles for change. Our personal problems and our relationship to them are the key to the world's transformation. We normally attempt to solve our inner turmoil by moving away from the solution to protect ourselves. Instead, we need to move toward understanding our false identification with our ego-driven personality. Real metamorphosis begins when we embrace our problems as agents of evolution and growth.

The current international political scene portrays this deeply embedded human crisis in a stark and powerful way. Millions of frustrated people are going to the streets and openly speaking their minds amidst a tsunami of emotional uproar. From Occupy Wall Street to the Arab Spring and the European economic crisis with its hefty austerity measures, people are showing their intolerance for ongoing authoritarian and outdated control measures. As we follow the unleashing eruptions from members from the entire human emotional spectrum, we also acknowledge that this revolutionary emerging voice can no longer be muted. As we shift our consciousness from the mind-orientated "functional" world into the center of our being, the heart, we inevitably have to get in touch with our emotions first. And given the fact that many of our emotions have been suppressed for thousands of years, the initial eruptive, potentially violent, scene may not be a pretty one! Getting in touch with our soul means simultaneously feeling our dormant pain.

Core Soul

To feel emotions is a beautiful experience as long as we strive to witness them and avoid becoming enmeshed with them. In general, feelings are of a neutral nature, sensations we perceive, whereas emotions are frequencies we react to, so often caused by people or circumstances. We are the ones who become reactive.

Feelings are sensations, which we may experience in any part of the body, like hot and cold or love and hate. Feelings express no judgment as they are directly born from the soul. They serve as pointers directing our choices throughout life. Feelings are essential in living a wholesome life. Emotions, on the other hand, are based on reactions and actions that involve someone or something outside us and are born from the realm of the ego-based personality. We can inflict violence, fueled by rage and anger, without actually feeling the frequency of sheer self-destruction. In fact, if we allowed ourselves to feel the depth of our rage, it would instantly come to a halt. When we stop, we have a space of communion in which we can experience stillness. It is this stillness of the very core alone that makes it possible for something different and new to emerge.

Emotions often have an eruptive character, whereas a feeling is a much calmer or fleeting experience. An emotion can also be stirred up if certain physical processes are interrupted, like breathing, nourishing, secreting, growing, or reproducing. For example, a hormonal imbalance, in women or men, can send a person into an emotional roller coaster of heightened intensity. One's conscious awareness and mindfulness about this explosive situation is the determining factor for whether we have the power to change its outcome. To embrace the soul, we have to understand how it feels to be reactive, how it feels to act recklessly, how it feels to blame our external world, and how it feels to witness our own self-limited distorted personality. We must become what we choose to experience in this world. The meeting of the soul is a quiet communion with one's feelings by going beyond the emotions.

Core Soul

As a holistic health physician, I have observed that most humans are willing to change unless life itself presses them against the wall to a place where all the exit holes are closed to them and where they are asked to give up control. Even when I strongly emphasize the importance of an organic, fresh diet, a healthy lifestyle, and cultivating a more positive relationship to life, the unfortunate truth is that a final breakthrough only occurs when someone is clearly challenged, either by disease, life-threatening pathology, or an emotional crisis. Change often requires this incredible wake-up call to push us into the direction of life-sustaining health and well-being.

If we could acknowledge the fact that these life-changing circumstances serve only as mirrors initiating the removal of what is blocked inside of us, we wouldn't keep insisting and fighting for our false delusions. It often boils down to fear, and fear caused by these blockages interrupts the flow of life. In cyclical fashion, if the internal flow of life contracts, the interrupted flow of energy affects the heart, which starts to display a weaker constitution, making it more and more susceptible to those lower vibrations, especially fear.

❦

Fear is the prime cause of the polarization of the scarred personality and the soul. In fact, it is the root of all prejudice and negative emotion. If you ask yourself what your purpose is in life after fulfilling all desires and dreams, you have to see that your spiritual evolution is founded in the removal of the blockages that cause that fear. To bypass or ignore fear we choose to focus on one particular aspect of an overall crisis, like my female patient who tormented herself over and over by saying: "If only he hadn't cheated on me! If only he hadn't left!" By selecting one distraction, we consciously manipulate ourselves to avoid seeing the overall picture and understanding the true learning experience of the situation. We then behave like human hamsters that run in self-created treadmills that lead to nowhere. By choosing to feed the distorted personality, we end up empty-handed indeed. The tendency to get drawn into our dramas is constant; it is the nature of the personality.

Core Soul

In Osho's words: "Don't move the way fear makes you move. Move the way love make you move. Move the way joy makes you move."

The willingness to go beyond our ego and raging personality therefore demands constant and daily attention.

There is nothing wrong in feeling emotions like fear, jealousy, or attraction. These are just frequencies and feeling such emotions is a normal attribute of being human. They do not, however, give us a specific identity. The purpose of evolution and growth is to learn how to witness these frequencies with awareness and mindfulness, rather than blindly react to them. In this way, all actions and thought patterns have a very different quality, one that is more free and boundless in nature.

Have you ever noticed that those people who unconsciously unleash their anger into the surrounding environment are the same ones who seem to get attacked or challenged by anger-provoking circumstances? This pattern feeds on the principle of similar resonance in the same way that we might prefer a certain radio station to another because its resonance matches our particular energetic frequency field. These situations are not as random as they might first appear, as they are in actuality serving as mirror images, presented to heal the person's core wound and overall perceptions.

Unfortunately, an intense and life-changing event of some kind is normally the precipitating factor for the person to wake up, to find himself, and break the continuous cycle of blame and justification for his inflicted misery. Unless he is willing to witness the center of the origin of his fear, the drama will continue to unfold in the same way that the collective drama in the world catches our attention each and every day. Your soul's request to you implies that you know yourself first in order to trust yourself again.

The first step in living life through your soul is becoming aware that your feelings are necessary and serve an essential and incredible purpose. Your feelings are a gift from your soul! We are only overwhelmed and thrown about by life when we resist understanding the core feelings of our emotions and manifested situations. To meet our soul and the soul of the world, we have to go beyond our emotions by witnessing our feelings within.

Core Soul

Pema Chödrön, author, teacher, and ordained nun of Tibetan Buddhism writes: "While we are sitting in meditation, we are simply exploring humanity and all of creation in the form of ourselves. We can become the world's greatest experts on anger, jealousy, and self-deprecation, as well as on joyfulness, clarity, and insight. Everything that human beings feel, we feel. We can become extremely wise and sensitive to all of humanity and the whole universe simply knowing ourselves, just as we are."

Most of our lives revolve around staying within our familiar comfort zones, our safety margins, and the space we know, reference, and identify with. Once you make the decision to work on your inner freedom it becomes impossible to remain in this "comfort" zone any longer because freedom and fear carry opposite energies and do not resonate together. The choice to live a liberated life from conditioned belief systems entails the daily commitment to leap beyond one's known self and to courageously break through known territories. To stay in the comfort zone implies you have accepted, and are perhaps resigned to living within a limited and confined space within yourself. Be courageous here. Harness all your energy, and then give it a try!

To live a courageous life doesn't mean boasting about your latest daring bungee-jump, your latest mountaintop conquest, or your six-figure salary. It also does not mean living a life where you deny yourself material possessions of the sort that may make you feel special, yet after all still ordinary. To courageously live on the edge, each and every day, demands our full attention in meeting and conquering our demons. While outer experiences might excite an adrenaline rush, a momentary mental or emotional fix for the personal ego, and certainly feels exciting, the lasting and true challenge requires the journey within. Only then can we live a truly brave and spontaneous life.

It is at this point that you will lose your desire to interact with the external world in an irresponsible manner in order to feed your internal boredom in hopes of filling the endless void. Your interest in collaborating with the outside world in a constructive and service-based manner, bypassing the ego-fueled tendencies, will surface. By turning your perception toward the light of your soul, you will be able to transform these self-limiting frequencies.

Core Soul

So often, our fear of taking the leap off an imaginary slippery edge imprisons us and binds us to self-created shackles. It might appear that the actual jump looks like an endless fall into an empty abyss with an envisioned negative outcome, yet in reality this small leap might be no more than six inches and require nothing more than a little encouragement and support. By limiting yourself, you are limiting the expansion of your consciousness and, indirectly, the consciousness of the world. In my view, we owe it to ourselves as well as to the planet to joyfully take that overdue leap into the unknown sooner than later. What hinders us here is our fear of change and the fear that something bad could happen as a result of this life-changing decision. When we truly start to awaken, however, we realize that we have caged ourselves and that this formerly accepted inner space has become an intolerably tight environment in which to live. We need to free ourselves from ourselves!

☙

I can wholeheartedly confirm that as my life began to change, what used to be my inner dance floor now looked like a tiny and limited space. Today, I can no longer feel comfortable living and expressing myself from that confined inner place. In fact, this daily challenge to overcome and go beyond my distorted self became an exhilarating and passionate endeavor, and now, each time I dare to conquer a bit more of my newfound inner territory, a surge of rejuvenated energy literally pours through my being, encouraging me to go even further next time.

Overcoming my initial hesitancy to step away from my fear and personal issues caused life to take on a very different outlook for me. The days are now dressed with an exciting flavor and a sense of joy as my own doing has birthed these feelings, rather than having them supplied to me by others or from the surrounding environment. More and more I enjoy feeling content with myself as I cherish the sweet, peaceful fragrance drifting gracefully through all parts of my life. I now understand what freedom is really about.

The cage that we project onto the world or in which we imprison ourselves is nothing more than a self-induced but imaginary realm of fear and discomfort. Once you decide to change this ingrained pattern by courageously moving toward your fears, it is natural to feel uncomfortable. When that happens, try to stay with your conviction to go beyond, to persevere and not to deviate from the chosen path. The feeling of discomfort is just another ego-based tool implemented in hopes that you will ditch your intention to overcome this inner hurdle. Going beyond the first hurdle will allow you to see how easy and exciting this new journey can be. To live a spiritual life entails the commitment to go beyond, no matter what it takes, each and every day, for the rest of your life. This journey is not a weekend practice, nor can it be done attending a weeklong seminar. It is your life; it is you.

As time goes by, you will realize what used to bother and upset you in the past has lost its validity and importance. As your focus turns inside, the sensation of feeling uncomfortable can now be associated to a feeling of resistance. Recognize this feeling as being afraid to take the next leap, rather than a statement about disserting your once upheld projections. To live a spiritual life means that you always live on the edge, never to return to your prior, always changing, inner comfort zone.

Paradoxically, while your inner world has dramatically changed, your external life might look quite settled—a stable profession, salary, family—but it is only when these external aspects become infused with your continuous courageous and passionate willingness to overcome your inner boundaries that your life will reflect a peaceful and soul-filled masterpiece.

Once you feel and allow yourself to move within your soul, you can really start to enjoy this boundless and unlimited space where there are no walls or limitations to confine the soul. It is exhausting to stay focused on keeping the inner known world's comfort zone intact, even when it is the foundation of your emotional misery and physical illness. If you could only see that your physical pain, your loneliness, your despair, your grief, or your frustration at work or home are all opportunities to challenge your perception and to come to the realization that your efforts to keep such "comforts" alive are destined to ultimately fail.

It is not life's events that cause problems or stress. It is our resistance to these events that cause this experience of life's misery. This mental muscle-effort to keep life in a fixed place requires an enormous amount of energy that leaves us drained and empty. What once was a draining experience in the past caused by a person or event has now become our own drainage process that keeps us from going beyond the small self to create a symbiotic partnership between the personality and the soul.

The idea that we have to hold onto something in order to be somebody now loses its credibility and meaning. The false sense of security we feel by holding onto negativity, past experiences, detrimental thoughts, and self-destructive behaviors reveals itself to be an inefficient system, one that only weakens the immune system and well-being. Hence, the perception of one's self-worth becomes about daring to live on the edge by living a spiritual life in a physical body, rather than about living a life in a physical body separate from the spiritual world. By becoming your own witness you will get to know your fears intimately, as well as your thoughts, your emotions, and your reactions. You will see that though you feel their existence and presence they are really not you after all. They never were. My suggestion is that each time you feel uncomfortable about somebody or a presenting situation, avoid trying to find a mental answer or solution based on the ego part of you, that part you consider your personality. Instead, try to witness yourself finding an objective answer by watching and observing your actions, thoughts, and emotions from a different perspective like an eagle from above. Start watching your distorted personality by feeling your distorted personality. As you pass through the golden door, the cloak of awareness will become your companion and lifelong dance partner.

☙

To switch from the identification of thoughts and emotions to a place free of judgment, criticism, and projections is the most rewarding and most challenging journey on which we can embark. Some will complain, "This is too hard!" And, while it is true that on this road you may experience yourself tearing apart, you will also experience a re-formation that permanently changes the way you see life. The journey is sure to be one that goes way beyond your wildest dreams! In facing the "unbearable" fears that drive you to think, feel, and act in a very limited way, your prison will collapse. As within, so without!

An inner peace and fulfilled contentment arises from the awareness that each and every day can be met with the knowing that there is no control, no safety zone, and no old belief system still operating. This peaceful feeling helps us stop blaming the outside world for its daily political failures and economic breakdowns by first turning the focus within. As long as we continue to entertain our old inner control mechanism, we will continue to attempt to control our external environment. This fundamental and profound change has to come from inside!

Michael A. Singer speaks on this theme in *The Untethered Soul*: "You must be willing to see that this need to protect yourself is where the entire personality comes from. It was created by building a mental and emotional structure to get away from the sense of fear. You are now standing face-to-face with the root of the psyche."

When you start living a spiritual life, you are different from everybody else. That which everybody else wants, you reject. That which everybody else resists, you welcome. You may even feel as if you don't fit into this world anymore. You have chosen your inner model to break, however, and you honor the experiences that cause you to feel uncomfortable or unsettled because you know this is part of growing.

Standing face-to-face with yourself is living from your core, the very depth of your being. Then freedom and liberation will not be just words, but a way of life. As you watch yourself change, you will master the art of "walking your talk." Then, you will begin to really live. The journey of becoming the soul takes us into the interior of ourselves, far into uncharted territories. Yet these territories are not unknown to the soul. When we speak of the "dark night of the soul," we often express our experience as one of despair, depression, and a feeling of losing oneself. But this moment of utter stillness and darkness is the very moment of true transformation. In this potentially seemingly unbearable moment in which you witness the unfolding spectrum of letting go of your fears and terror they will begin to fade. Without your nurturing, without your identification with them, they lose all power. The extent of our falsely perceived separation and division within and on the planet without reflects the extent of the suffering we will incur. Remember, every lotus flower rises out of the depth of the mud in which it burrows.

Life is all about balance in movement. In this soul-orientated journey, there is also a fine balance between focusing too much on the soul or not at all. If we turn too much inward, we create the danger of isolating ourselves from the whole, an effort that results in separation of the present moment and reality. Let us not get too caught up in our dream analysis, therefore, or the ongoing interpretation of our distorted personalities, as doing so can tempt us to unconsciously start identifying with our inner content. The real soul doesn't carry any content at all; it is boundless spaciousness and everything in nothingness. When we succumb to focusing on content we continue to resist experiencing the soul.

To clarify, the "I" and the ego are not the same. Ego is formed from past experiences that create a false kind of self. The "I" is a higher form of self, the part of you that is more fluid and creative and resonates with the future. We might envision how each "I" connects each individual soul with the soul of the world.

༄

Rudolph Steiner, an Austrian philosopher, social reformer, architect, and founder of anthroposophy speaks about the soul in this way: "The 'I' is an aspect of the soul—not the soul life of the past, but the soul's participation in the future."

Once you start cultivating your individual interrelationship with your soul and its spiritual purpose, you feel inspired to connect with the world outside in a different way. Your sensitivity will heighten, all of your senses stimulated to transform your life into a sensual experience. Touch, sight, taste, smell, and hearing become your spiritual tools rather than mere anatomical features. You will find yourself expanding beyond your physical boundaries by sensing everything around you, in the world and beyond. You become One with What Is!

Core Soul

In *Love and the Soul* Robert Sardello, co-director of the School of Spiritual Psychology, points out: "Soul is not an entity but an activity. Paradoxically, in discovering that true individuality of soul is not something one has but something one must create and in taking up this task, spiritual culture forms from moment to moment. We are what we make and the moment we stop soul-making we are less than what we could be."

☙

Your dance has changed! Your movements become more fluid, your body turns and sways with the rhythm of your soul rather than only to the sound of the music. In fact, in this very moment, it doesn't matter anymore if the music plays or not, as you are dancing to the sound of your soul.

You can transcend all negativity when you realize that the only power it has over you is your belief in it. As you experience this truth about yourself you are set free.

—Eileen Caddy

Ensouled Body Dances with Embodied Soul

> Your vision will become clear only when you look into your heart.
> Who looks outside ... dreams; who looks inside ... awakens.
>
> —Carl Gustav Jung

As we turn our dance more and more within, the body doesn't feel the need so much anymore to move by itself, but prefers to synchronize its movement to the voice inside. It recognizes the opportunity in expanding from within to without by deeply feeling the fullness of life with all its senses. The best way to allow your feelings to be present is by getting in touch with Nature. So, let's take a walk!

You are enjoying a walk through a wheat field on a late summer afternoon. The air is still filled with the heat of the sun, the fluffy white clouds are spread across the horizon, and in the far distance you are aware of the presence of some farm life. As you stand in the midst of the track lines created by man's agricultural machineries' burrowing, you are reminded of deep grooves on a weathered old farmer's face. Your breath comes to a momentary halt while taking in this extraordinary moment. You feel compelled to stretch out both your arms to either side of you to touch the amber waves of thigh-high grains of golden wheat. You close your eyes and start walking with all your senses wide open. Your ears take in the crushing sound of the already flattened stalks as each of your shoes brushes their skin. Your face feels the slight *breeze that carries the scent of the late summer farm life. As your hands glide over countless wheat crowns and feel the bristly material that protects the wheat kernel, you are reminded of a rough beard on a young man's face. Simultaneously, a thought comes into your mind that this bristly beard might protect the wheat from inclement weather conditions. How wonderful of Nature to think that way.*

As you keep walking, you feel the strong and sturdy stems firmly supporting the stalks' precious heads. Although they are hollow and will become straw after the kernel is harvested, you are amazed at their powerful presence. While tuning into your experience, you become aware of the main purpose of the wheat root that gathers nourishment from the soil to allow the plant to grow strong and healthy, giving us its life-promoting building blocks. Right now, you are feeling life and you are dancing with Nature.

☙

This description of a wheat stalk is very fresh in my mind, as only a few months ago I walked through such a field in the English countryside to enjoy my meditation in a crop circle. This was my chance to experience just how elaborate these patterns of geometric shapes are. Though some areas of grain are tamped down and others are left intact, the edge between the two is so clean it appears to be created with a machine—or by a non-human energy. I noticed that even though the stalks were bent, they remained undamaged.

As I contemplated the bent stalks in the field more closely, I couldn't help notice the precision of all the design. As I tuned into the presence of the circles, I felt strongly that an outer-world laser beam, like the ones we might use in microsurgeries today yet much bigger in size and power must be responsible for these formations. The wheat stalks, heavily pressed down into the ground, leave the impression that a massive weight, perhaps as heavy as concrete, has been applied to flatten the designated areas. In my meditation, I asked for the purpose of these incredible shapes without trying to interpret or analyze their meaning. As I quieted myself, I immediately received the answer: Angelika, the meaning and purpose of it all is this: you have to love yourself more and more and more, go to a place you have never gone before and that you have never imagined exists within yourself. Only then will you become an active participant and an active partner in the change of this New World.

The message was simple, direct, and yet deeply profound. As I integrated my experience as the day went on, I asked myself: Which aspect in my life can receive more love? and received a clear reply: My body.

Since that day in the crop circle, I have chosen to adapt my diet to consist of more raw and fresh foods and have cultivated an even more refined sense of listening to my body. You might say that my body took on the role of the crop circle, both able to activate itself and serve as the catalyst for existential transmissions. I always wondered why so many crop circles consistently appear in the county of Wiltshire, situated in the southwest of England. Having engaged with the people there, I now know why. The inhabitants' emotional hearts shape and nurture their perception of their surroundings and life. The landscape has drawn to itself farmers who care deeply about the land, their animals, and their people.

Communion with the body serves as a direct entrance to the soul as the body is the instrument of the soul. The sweet singing of a well-played violin, the deeply penetrating piano concerto, or the pulsating sound of an electric guitar can only be birthed by its player. It is the musician's emotions and connection to his or her soul that facilitates the elegance and mastery of the instrument. The emotional frequencies transmitted into the instrument come through choices about which feelings the musician wants to express through the music. The musician feels the music and so do we, the ones receiving this exquisite frequency. The body serves as a vehicle that houses the soul.

Core Soul

During this global birthing process in co-creating a collective humanity, we are asked to leave our identification with our belief systems behind, to feel more and allow our feelings to point us in the direction beyond those belief systems. We know that common crisis situations often catapult us into emotional realms and that being in those realms affect the body, which then manifests symptoms of pain and discomfort. These symptoms are our guide into the deeper parts of ourselves. Pain by itself is really just a sensation, but the experience of being in pain or living with pain with all its attached thoughts makes this experience very real. We are given these symptoms and sensations as keys to open the doors to a more liberated and authentic Self. In my personal story, pain became my demon and my liberator at the same time as I experienced and then shifted both the physical and emotional pain.

Pain is an initiator, the priest or priestess with the wisdom and power to emancipate us from our identification with the body that lives with it. To free yourself from pain, you will have to go through it, as paradoxical as that sounds. Eckhart Tolle, best-selling author and philosopher, perfectly describes this part of ourselves as the "pain-body," because we literally give it an identity and invite it to live separately but alongside us.

Let's look at the individual who desires to connect with his feelings and open up his heart, yet is having a difficult time of it. When an outside situation presents itself that scratches on the inner world of his feelings, he chooses to act coldly indifferent, and somehow "above" his feelings. He would rather avoid getting in touch with how he feels than delve more deeply into these feelings. Soon, his abrupt and detached actions stir up a deep-seated, unresolved belief system of rejection in his spouse (or friend or colleague). His spouse, who now feels rejected, experiences emotional pain, which after some time manifests in the physical symptom of stomach pain (or other symptomatology indicating the mind and body are in pain). Neither of these people are acting from a fundamental place of truth as each is only reacting to a deeply ingrained belief system that insists they avoid feeling, pain, and rejection at all cost. As both parties identify with their core wounds as if they were real and unmovable, rather than feel through the wounds as manifestations of their distorted perception of self and other, a very confused and misunderstood relationship results. On a larger scale, these personal and collective false perceptions are the culprit behind the dividing collective humanity today.

To feel, accept, and reclaim your core wound is the first step to walking through the veil of false perception. In owning the possibility that your reoccurring backache might have something to do with the general lack of support in your life or that your frequent asthma attacks, despite all the medications, might stem from a deep-seated anxiety or panic that constricts your breathing capacity, or that your sky-rocketing blood pressure might be related to your stressful relationship with your spouse, you clarify your position. Will you be controlled by your physical symptoms and false perceptions—or live a life free of projections?

Pain and physical ailments may be the soul's way of quieting the stubborn ego and asking you to reflect on this process. If we can resist the temptation to sedate the experience of pain through medication, emotional suppression, and/or complete denial, we can become our own midwife in birthing the accumulated and lifeless energy blocks in order to serve the healing of the soul. It is really a phenomenal process when the body becomes the entrance to the soul, rather than simply a mechanical device with a separate existence.

When we are unable to let go or detach ourselves from our daily events they eventually accumulate and become stagnant, like a murky pool of water in the body. Feelings are like waves, currents that come and go, briefly kissing the shore and then quickly retreating into the vastness of the ocean. Holding onto outworn emotional patterns only adds to the already decaying debris within.

Any current, from the electrical to the spiritual, needs to move, to find an outlet in order to regenerate its life with vibrant energy. No movement is equal to congested energy, which is ultimately the cause of illness. When feelings are suppressed or denied, the dormant, frustrated energy, in need of movement, contacts the mind first. This is why we so often go into a mental frenzy after we've been hurt, betrayed, or mistreated. We mentally argue, rectify, and negotiate in order to release the initially censored energy via our thought processes. If we still can't find a resolution using our mind, which is most often the case, we end up more frustrated and stir up further emotional chaos.

The energy current, still searching for an outlet, now rages within the body like a trapped snake trying to find the way out. Due to the resistance to the force of change, the most vulnerable way out is to the heart, which will carry the accumulated emotional load. We then either try to push these energies away from us or try to hold onto them because we feel attracted to them. The primal desire provoked by a deeply instinctual need, the yearning to connect the body and soul, is hereby interrupted. As long as we resist the natural rhythm and flow of our feelings, we restrict the flow of the vital force with its unlimited and renewable energy supply within.

Real growth, which includes breaking away from these internal mind-traps, takes place when we fully commit ourselves to deal with pain that is often based on fear alone. The mental, emotional, and/or physical pain has to be faced in order to welcome the core of the individual, the true Self. The expressions of and actions fueled by the resistance to one's personal emotional or physical pain penetrate every aspect of our life. We can't run away from this pain, nor can we disguise it with our skilled manipulating and selfish mind games. We are notoriously adept at keeping ourselves occupied, hiding behind a wall of false confidence, trying to prove ourselves in order to be liked, locking ourselves away in depression, or controlling ourselves and others in order to avoid the real issue: the pain.

The time has come for us to recognize and experience the collapse of these operating systems now that they are fully exposed and found to be unacceptable to the soul. Our hearts are crying out for individual liberation as well as for the liberation of the world. Even if this path to facing your inner demons initially scares you to death, you cannot run away from it. If you continue to run away from the truth, life will present you with ever more challenging tests on the same reoccurring themes. Avoidance only incites the stomach ulcer—that burning and illuminating voice that speaks to you by reminding you of your underlying emotional pain based on the feeling that you were not cared for or nurtured.

Core Soul

As the body serves us as an instrument of the soul, we start to experience elevated sensations like joy and love, which in the context of this new consciousness take on very different roles and can be seen as existential needs, rather than fleeting feelings. Rather than seeing them as "good feelings," we see them emerge as guides pointing us to confirm our choices and expressions in life. When we feel joyful and give or receive love, the body is living the visible expression of the soul.

ॐ

In the past, few people dared to go to this place of inner freedom, a privilege mostly reserved for enlightened spiritual masters or highly awakened humans who committed themselves to the spiritual path. This is the very reason we consult and visit these masters, as they remind us to re-kindle the flame of a purposeful and soulful life again. To learn from a master is admirable, yet every true master will send his disciple out in the world, usually after a period of 12 years of training, to integrate and apply the many lessons learned.

The Age of Aquarius, denoting either the current (or upcoming, depending on the calculation) astrological age, emphasizes the need for all of us to become our own masters and be willing to live a masterfull life, as so many saints and enlightened beings have done before us. This new paradigm in consciousness requests our full attention to step up to the challenge. Our goal is to become living spiritual masters within ourselves, without fostering co-dependence on external personified leaders.

The time has come to create a life based on maturity, integrity, and a chosen commitment to free one's self! Once you live your authentic life, free of self-imposed preferences and conditioning, you will see that this unlimited space of feeling free always has been very close to you, in fact much nearer than you initially thought. Avoiding the pain doesn't work anymore. To face and transform the pain is the price for freedom! We are born to transform; it is the very purpose of our life. To resist this emerging force means resisting life itself. The path and form of transformation may look and feel very different for each of us. Certainly there is no manual to follow. But this does not mean it will be easy to keep from criticizing or judging each other. With that said, there are a number of basic concepts or ingredients required to facilitate this change, the most significant being the release from fear as portrayed by letting go of long worn-out belief systems, the resistance to bodily sensations, and the courageous willingness to step through or behind the veil of delusions to the needed awareness. These factors will accompany the individual to the point where he or she will be able to take the leap of faith quite easily. In fact, the entire spectrum of the psyche's building blocks, both the darker and lighter aspects, brings forth the true form of Self.

It is a bit like baking a loaf of bread. For the yeast to rise the dough needs food in the form of warmth and moisture. Only then can it convert from flour (sugar and starch) through the fermentation process into carbon dioxide and alcohol. The totality of all the ingredients is needed to give birth to a form, the loaf of bread. The true beauty of this analogy is evident when we compare it to the way our worst feared images and perceptions need to reform just like the dough into a new structure. Then the totality of all our aspects becomes the building blocks for our personal, as well as planetary, transformation. Each of those aspects, especially the ones we have ignored and suppressed, need examination for us to take that necessary leap in freeing and fulfilling our Self. The beauty of welcoming the entire spectrum of emotions and delusions manifests in the illumination of the soul.

By upholding false perceptions, we polarize the body from the soul. By surrendering to ourselves, we are reborn to our authentic Self, without attachment to any external religious institution or co-dependent authority figures. This process should not be seen and understood as the physical death, but the death of the ego only, that part of us that has divorced the body from the soul. This daily "dying" process can then become the most exquisite and sweet gift we give ourselves each day.

When I am faced with challenging situations, I often find peace and encouragement in attending a sacred ceremony, a sweat lodge, a meditation circle, or simply by repeating a mindful prayer, or setting some time aside to consciously meet this demanding moment in reverence and sanctity. By giving conscious attention to the self, we continuously adjust the distorted personality with regard to the soul, scraping away, a little more of the hidden jewel within the block of marble each and every time. By feeling the resistance, as well as the opening and willingness to change, we will also feel our emotional heart.

🙦

The heart is accustomed to the movement of giving and receiving. While physical blood flows through its chambers, it either receives oxygenated blood or sends away deoxygenated blood. The heart is also well equipped in releasing and receiving feelings like the waves crashing onto and away from the shore, naturally following a rhythm of ebb and flow. The need to protect or defend the heart, either from oneself or the outside, only interferes with this natural rhythm. To trust one's self requires a deep intimate relationship with the emotional and spiritual heart. This lasting and intimate relationship with Self can only flourish if the shields of protection are courageously removed. As we witness the ebb and flow of fleeting sensations, of images, thoughts, and emotions, it is like watching a film passing in front of the eyes because we can detach ourselves from its context and from identifying with it. In this way we can achieve more peaceful neutrality. To dance with an open heart changes the journey of dancing with the soul to a much sweeter experience. This sense of inner equilibrium becomes the basis for the capacity to trust.

[If you are interested in learning about belief systems, which are often passed on by birth and registered in astrological natal charts, I highly recommend the book *Astrology for the Soul* by Jan Spiller. In this book, the placement of the North Node of the astrological chart indicates qualities of one's belief system and the destiny of his chosen life. You do not have to be an astrologer to understand this book, as time charts guide the reader to his or her personal core issue.]

Let's have a closer look what the physical and emotional heart is really about. Most of us believe that the heart acts as a pump to circulate blood and generate pressure waves throughout the body. This is the standard medical version to describe the heart as an organ. But it is also an outdated way of looking at the heart, which is clearly much more than a muscular pump. Scientific studies enlighten us that the heart is like an electromagnetic generator with a wide spectrum of electromagnetic frequencies, as well as a facilitator of hormones, similar to all our other endocrine glands. The heart is intimately connected to the central nervous system and therefore acts like a brain on its own. Yes, you read correctly: the heart is a brain—and much better equipped than the organ that is the "actual" brain as we know it.

The heart takes care of multiple chemical processes. It also sends information regarding body temperature and rising and falling blood pressure to the brain and the rest of the body. All these heart-related processes not only affect physiological functions, but also deeply influence consciousness relative to how we think and feel.

This incredible and majestic muscle beats 100,000 times a day, 40 million times a year, and about 3 billion times throughout an average lifespan. Two gallons of blood per minute, or 100 gallons an hour, journey through all the bodily vessels in the human body. The heart oversees this network of vessels, which make up this complex and intricate circulatory system. It is estimated that if all of the vessels were laid end to end they would have a length of 60,000 miles, more than twice the circumference of the Earth. The heart is an incredible and mind-blowing divine invention, not simply a mechanical instrument as seen by the Newtonian model.

The heart, as an organ, doesn't have the capacity to circulate so much blood throughout the body; instead it uses its capacity to hold the space for the blood in order to allow it to continue its circulatory process. The blood actually moves by its own accord, confined by a system that acts like the edges of a riverbed. Scientific studies have revealed that the blood in chicken embryos starts to flow before the heart is developed enough to act as its pump!

Today, we know that blood itself is composed of two streams that spiral around one another toward one common goal. The streams don't flow at the same speed and can vary significantly. The individuality of each stream is the reason for the fluctuating temperature within the blood. As these two streams weave and turn into each other like a spiraling DNA strand, their center, or core, is completely empty, a space of nothingness. The composition of the blood more or less resembles a vortex circling around the space of vacuum. This vacuum serves as an essential part in producing the vortex itself. What we call "blood pressure" does not actually relate to the pumping action of the heart, but solely to the movement of the spiraling blood itself.

In Nature, our primal design of creation can be traced back to the spiral. The spiral is one of the oldest and most enigmatic sacred images known. It appears encoded in plants, leaves, flowers, fruits, and seed patterns; in animals, like fish and cetaceans; in musical harmonies; and throughout Earthly and galactic structures. It is also seen in proportional ratios in the well-known Fibonacci sequence of numbers and in the Nautilus shell, the spiraling pattern of a cauliflower, or the movement of draining water or the rotating newborn pushing itself through its birthing canal. Nature often appears to be founded on this core energy-creating pattern that offers itself as the visual manifestation for the evolution of life. This double spiral, as seen in the blood or in the DNA strand, creates an environment of natural boundaries without unnecessary rigidity or tension.

Throughout our history, the greatest damage we've perpetrated on our streams and rivers is straightening out their boundaries and interfering with their natural rhythm and meandering movements. This mindless, industrialized human intervention not only affects all life, civilized or animal, near the trapped water, but also decreases the energy and electrical potential of the water itself. Water is alive just as blood is alive. Both need to regenerate by spiraling in a vortex-like motion, similar to the funnel of a tornado. Blood needs to move, twirl, and dance around its core!

The blood is not propelled by its pressure, but rather moves with its own biological momentum and with its own intrinsic flow of pattern.
—Ralph Marinelli, Director of Rudolf Steiner Research Center

Even the single elements within blood, the blood cells, display this centrifugal action by spinning around their own axis of rotation. This rotating energy field emanates from the body through consciousness and all existence.

Core Soul

Rudolph Steiner's speaks about the heart: "The heart is not a pump! I have often said this; it is rather an organ for sensing or registering the activity of the tissue fluid. The heart is moved by the circulation of the blood; it is not the pumping action of the heart that moves the blood. Just as the thermometer is nothing more than an instrument for registering the degree of heat or cold, so your heart is like an apparatus for registering what takes place in the circulation and what flows into this form, the metabolic system."

Few of us know that the heart produces at least five different hormones (ANF, CNP, BNF, HPVD, CGRP) that have a broad impact on the heart, the brain, and the overall body. What is most interesting is that the hormones ANF, CNP and BNF all strongly impact the hippocampus and integrated functions of the central nervous system, which influences learning and memory as well as the ability to take action in a new environment. The hippocampus is a major component of the brain of humans and other vertebrates and belongs to the limbic system. The hippocampus plays an important role in consolidating information in short-term and long-term memory processes and in spatial navigation.

Produced by the heart and released into the bloodstream, such hormones profoundly affect how and what we learn, how we remember, and how well we remember. The more hormones are produced, the better we remember and the better we learn.

In fact, the heart is directly wired into the central nervous system and interconnected with the brain. The heart also expresses its own memory, as it possesses the same kind of neurons as the brain. As in those cases with people who receive heart transplants and take on the behaviors of the individual whose heart they now house, though the heart may initially be foreign to the recipient, the implanted heart's memory banks clearly affect the perception and consciousness of its new owner.

Just as the heart and brain are in constant communication with each other to share valuable information, so are the physiological functions and cellular behaviors. Remember, the environment changes the behavior of the cells.

Core Soul

Any information that flows through the body will impact the heart first, and then will flow to the brain only after the heart has perceived it. This means that life experiences filter through the heart first. The heart analyzes the information, thinking it through before sending the compiled data to the brain for further processing. Feelings and emotional sensations hereby serve as direct indicators of the quality of thought processes and actions. Each neuron in the brain changes its frequencies in response to the signals received by each heartbeat.

As the brain sends back processed information to the heart, it re-evaluates it to decide whether or not the ideas are suited to the totality of the individual. It does not automatically obey the brain's messages, but interprets the information based on its emotional status. The heart has its own logic with its inherent intelligent language. As the heart and brain continuously communicate with each other they should both be viewed as deciding influences over which actions are beneficial to our physical functioning and well-being.

The heart isn't only responding to what's going on inside the body, but consciously affecting our exterior world to a large degree. Its measurable electromagnetic field touches the electromagnetic field of every living organism, inviting the possibility of vital energy exchanges. This perspective allows us to see the heart as an organ of perception. A coherent heart, capable of thinking and expressing itself in a clear and consistent manner, not only affects our brain wave patterns, but also the patterns of any living thing, plant or animal, that comes in close proximity or contact with us.

Radiating a heart-coherent field filled with caring and loving energy inspires other living creations to respond to the out-pouring of energy. Those affected will become more open and connected with themselves and the world at large... and so on. Did you know that the heart's electromagnetic field, measured with magnetic field meters, is about 5,000 times more powerful than that created by the brain? This fact in itself should galvanize us to start living from the center of our heart, rather than the faculty of mind.

The electromagnetic field produced by the heart extends into space in a spherical shape around the body, flowing out and returning in an endless stream. The electromagnetic field of the Earth with its South and North magnetic poles displays a similar pattern to the heart's vibrational field, continuously receiving and sending energy to all living beings as generated by its ever-unfolding information. This spherical formation is also referred to as the torus, the mathematical term for a donut shape or a circle with a smaller hole in the middle that receives and emanates frequencies.

The body, on a smaller scale, functions like a radio transmitter for incoming frequencies as well as out-streaming vibrations that flow into its environment. In fact, the whole body is sweetly embraced by the electromagnetic field generated by the heart. This spherical shape of moving energy (the torus) isn't a fixed form, but flexible in nature and constantly shifting its structure according to the incoming information it receives from internal and external sources. All incoming information is distributed throughout the body via the bloodstream, which then conducts electromagnetic impulses throughout the body. What comes into your body affects your blood and ultimately the behavior of your cells.

If we continue to support the idea that the body is separated from the soul and the world from its planetary soul, we only deprive ourselves of vital life-forming energy resources. We are connected with the soul through the body, just as our body and soul are connected with the soul of the world by their participation in it.

Bruce Lipton and Steve Bhaerman writes in his latest book *Spontaneous Evolution*: "Science suggests that the next stage of human evolution will be marked by awareness that we are all interdependent cells within the super-organism called humanity."

In this context homeopathy is still widely misunderstood regarding its deeply transformative science and application. The effectiveness of homeopathy is founded on the stimulation of one's own vital force, on the very vibration that keeps you alive. New discoveries in physics are beginning to explain this phenomenon. One theory states that succussion, the shaking of a chosen substance, creates an electromechanical pattern, and that this pattern, stored in a diluted liquid of water and alcohol, spreads like liquid crystals through the body's own water. Another hypothesis suggests that the dilution process triggers an electromagnetic imprinting that directly affects the body's electromagnetic field. As we start to merge our evolving consciousness with a more direct and intimate relationship with the body, we will hopefully also begin appreciating the brilliance of homeopathy. I look forward to a time when this field is fully incorporated in the New World as a mainstream form of medicine existing in parallel with allopathic medicine. It is my belief that any form of medicine based on vibrational healing must be the most effective and have the most lasting medicinal benefit in that it correlates to the vibrational body of the person and the planet.

Until we open our hearts and minds to the fundamental understanding that we are composed of living energy formations that best respond to vibrational healing modalities, our bodies will only be offered limited opportunities to recover from destructive diseases.

☙

Lee Harris, healer, energy teacher, dear friend, and author of *Energy Speaks* expresses the information about our planet via his channeled transmission in these terms: "Heart energy is rising on the planet right now. What is also rising is the ability for all of us to see energy. We are all being allowed to see beyond the veil whether that is the energy of a person, the energy of a place or the energy of a situation. Energy drives everything we do. Energy is the driving force behind our choices, our relationships, our interactions, how we feel and how we move on any given day. The energy of the heart is the core of our energetic being, our energetic force, our energetic expression embodies in human form."

Our heart can be seen as an open-energy system that needs to interact with other energy forms. As the heart decodes and encodes information, it also generates and delivers varying waves of information directly to the brain, which are then distributed to the rest of the body. Your heart is a complex and ingenious creation! Due to its sensory capacity, it is hypersensitive to feelings. Emotions, from love to hate, but particular negative-based frequencies, affect its electromagnetic field and its spherically shaped formation of outgoing energy flow. Anybody who comes close to this electromagnetic energy field, whether a rock, animal, or human, will feel that energy as well, like ripples spreading over the surface of a pond after a stone has been thrown in. We are all affected and influenced by our exterior and interior energy fields.

To truly feel our emotions is the key to this experience that leads us to the soul. It may appear that we are capable of feeling, yet many of us feel inclined to either suppress or deny these potential emotions. Allowing yourself to feel your love, anger, jealousy, or restlessness implies that you are giving yourself permission to let the feeling be present in yourself without necessarily identifying with or reacting to it. Witnessing your feelings by fully acknowledging them and simultaneously cultivating a kind of neutrality toward them is the first step to becoming the conscious creator of a coherent electromagnetic field generated by your heart. In this manner, your brain and nervous system will be influenced and calibrated in a coherent way, allowing you to live a coherent life.

The rhythm and dance of the heart influences the general rhythm of the body and, on a larger scale, the world. The heart, with its rhythmic beating and cognitive and emotional functions, not only influence the brain but the central and autonomic nervous systems. Your emotions are therefore reflected in the patterns of the rhythm of your heart. Your excitement, the fluttering of your heart, nervousness, joy, and fear are all registered in the rhythm of your heart's dance movements. And these changes in rhythm influence its overall electromagnetic field.

༄

We know that heart disease, next to colon cancer, is the number-one killer in the U.S. today. Rather than brutally deforming the heart with stents, artificial valves, mechanical devices, and an arsenal of drugs, I advocate a new approach. How about healing the heart with the coherent electromagnetic field generated by the patient himself along with the application of vibrational devices that feed the incoming information with a coherent frequency? Let's base our treatment on healing, rather than on treatments that deplete the heart's energetic field.

Just a few days ago, I came across a newspaper article describing how a 23-year-old man had stunned his medical team when his deficient heart appeared to mend itself after the doctors had made the decision to perform a transplant. The man was suffering from an inflammation of the heart muscle caused by acute myocarditis, which had left the vital organ barely functioning, but had a blood infection that threatened the doctors' ability to proceed with the transplant. As the patient was in a medically induced coma the doctors soon decided the transplant would be too risky.

Suddenly the young man's blood pressure began to stabilize. The doctors looked on, amazed, as his heart began to heal itself, to beat on its own—and without intervention. When the doctors reassessed with new tests they were shocked to find that the patient's left heart chamber had indeed begun the healing process without aid of any kind. During this man's hospital stay, his family and friends had started a prayer chain with daily posted updates on a public website. The page attracted more than 30,000 visitors and 1,100 comments. Through an e-mail blast, a staggering number of 3,000 families started to pray for the young man's complete and smooth recovery. The young man's parents attributed his recovery to the power of prayer.

Prayer or any conscious set intention creates a frequency, a living current, which not only affects the electromagnetic heart field of the person praying, but the recipient of the healing frequency, whose own electromagnetic heart field receives and decodes the incoming information for its own needed healing purpose.

When the heart becomes "coherent," the brain immediately begins to respond. Then the senseless chattering of the addictive thought processes quiet down. This allows us to step away from the small self by embracing the soulful heart. It is when we shift our consciousness into the brain rather than the heart, which guides the brain, that we encourage the disconnection of body and soul.

In *The Secret Teachings of Plants* Stephen Buhner, an Earth Poet and senior researcher for the Foundation for Gaian Studies writes: "Heart coherence begins when the location of consciousness is shifted from the brain to the heart, either through focus on the heart itself or on external sensory cues and how they feel."

The story of how the young man's heart healed "on its own" clearly demonstrates us how the heart's electromagnetic field can influence physical healing. Studies have also shown that an increased heart-brain coherence directly influences physical health. Through the body's production of Immunoglobulin A, many diseases like arrhythmia, mitral valve prolapse, congestive heart failure, asthma, diabetes, fatigue, autoimmune conditions, autonomic nervous system exhaustion, anxiety, depression, AIDS, and post-traumatic stress disorders are greatly improved and re-balanced. One study found that high blood pressure alone could be significantly lowered within six months without medication of any kind when heart coherence was cultivated. People who experience panic or anxiety attacks and depression also report great improvement as they synchronize the messages from their brains with those of their hearts.

The more we focus on our daily reactions of anger, rage, or frustration, the more incoherent our heart's electromagnetic field becomes. This incoherence affects the entire physical body. How can we consciously participate in or work with our emotions without getting too deeply involved? I personally have found the Buddhist Meditation called Tonglen very beneficial. This ancient practice from Tibet teaches us how to open the heart by cultivating love and kindness toward Self and others. This powerful meditation can bring about a transformation in the way we perceive others and the world around us. You can use Tonglen anytime during the day to get in touch with your heart, your deepest Self, and those around you.

Tonglen Meditation

Find a comfortable place and take a few minutes out of your busy life schedule. This place can be found on a park bench, in your office, even in your bathroom or a quiet corner of your favorite café. If you want to find a peaceful place, you'll find it! This quiet moment will provide you with the needed space of undisturbed silence and peace to allow your feelings to be heard. Remember to switch off your cell phone and prepare yourself to spend some time with yourself only.

Core Soul

Invite your most uncomfortable issue in your life to surface. Feel which one is the one that incites your reaction the most or that you most want to deny. Take a deep breath in... beyond the boundaries of your skin, beyond the organized structure of your bones... and open your heart. Now allow the uncomfortable feeling to be taken up by your breath until it finally rests in your heart. As you breathe in this heavy, dark, red, hot energy, give it permission to sweetly reside, even just for a brief moment, in your big and expanded heart. With each following in-breath, imagine the walls of your heart pushing outwards, each time a little more, continuing to create more space while welcoming your temporary emotional block. Breathe in your physical pain, your deep-seated grief, your churning anger, your experience of being betrayed that never seems to go away, or your shame, your guilt, or your poisonous jealousy ... breathe it all in and let it sit in the garden of your heart. Just let it be! Don't analyze it or judge it. Just welcome it as a temporary guest within you. Don't be afraid, the guest will not stay, it is only a guest and it will leave your safe garden shortly.

As your in-breath reaches the top of your lungs, slowly start to exhale by sending out this dark and heavy frequency, now transformed into pure light. It may be a bluish, cooling color now as it moves into the external world. See this brilliant fresh light radiating out in all directions, completely leaving your body by leaving no trace behind. Synchronize your breathing with the dark energy coming in and the cool, refreshing energy going out.

Repeat this process as long as you need to, until you feel your heart is relaxed enough to move on. Be courageous; you owe it to yourself. Take a full in-breath and then let go. Whenever your lungs are fully expanded, you can't hold onto anything anymore, as you already feel full from the inside. Once you have invited into your open heart your seemingly worst enemy, relax. Continue to completely empty yourself out, even if it takes several attempts to reach this point.

If your body starts to respond with sensations like trembling or feeling that you can't breathe or tears begin running down your cheeks, do not interfere with this moment of release. Give your body the chance to participate in its own cleansing process. You are safe and your soul wants you to release. During this moment of reclaiming your ability to feel and think with your heart, you will also get in touch with other dormant and accumulated emotional scar tissues, mostly related to past wounds. As you allow your heart to open to these hidden treasures within, you begin to strip away the old scars as well. This process allows the heart to soften and become flexible again, facilitating the potentiality to use it as an invaluable tool and as an organ of perception.

When you have fully emptied yourself, continue to expand your vision by focusing on a loved one or a family member who is in need of some help. This individual may simply be going through a difficult time or perhaps triggers you in some way. Breathe in his or her pain, grief, depression, or whatever you feel is connected with this person and then slowly let it go, completely and in all directions.

When you feel you are ready to move on, focus on all the people in the world who experience pain, violence, starvation, or other personally difficult situations. This meditation allows you to acknowledge your own suffering and that of others, as well as the feeling of sending it back in love and peace. Each and every day, we see suffering in our daily lives. Our child has a bad day at school, a friend struggles with physical pain, a co-worker gets fired, or someone you know is burdened with a long-standing depression. The amount of pain in the world often feels overwhelming and there are days were I too couldn't watch another news clip.

By allowing uncomfortable feelings related to both personal and worldly issues to just be . . . to be present without interference, to be witnessed in all their fullness, you will not only heal your mental, emotional, or physical pain, but also contribute to the energetic shift of the world. As your electromagnetic field of your heart starts to align itself in a coherent pattern, so will the electromagnetic field of the environment around you.

ॐ

If we commit ourselves to grow and evolve, we are always going to be stepping out of our comfort zone. Allowing the distorted personality to be present by giving it temporary permission to be with its host accomplishes the same thing. Exploring new dimensions in the perception of life can enhance the way we perceive information and bring a brighter and more peaceful quality into our lives.

To feel means to truly allow feelings to be present. This is an act of embracing and acknowledging them without forcing any preconceived notions onto their existence and expression. Challenging preconceived notions, realities, stories, and ideas frees us and heals us of their energetic hold. We tend to shy away from these feelings, avoiding them by sitting for hours in front of the TV or drowning our hearts in alcohol or prescription and recreational drugs. But these actions only serve to temporarily dampen their impact; the more we push them down, the more they are sure to affect us. To be free requires we embrace the feelings and lose the story—the content of the experience.

Labeling an emotion for quality, depth, and content does not mean we are not still chained to the personality. The key is to feel your anger, but maintain a critical or rectifying attitude about it so you do not allow it to be felt in its entirety. It is possible to spend a lifetime with our thoughts chasing their own tails without ever dipping into the true source of the emotions we experience. Your body will likely register the impact of the emotion through sensations like inflammation, cramped muscles, or increased saliva in the mouth—but this does not mean you are truly feeling the full spectrum of the anger's emotional frequency. If we give ourselves permission to fully feel the anger by witnessing the nature of that anger from an impersonal point of view, however, its power will immediately subside, fizzling out like a wet match.

So, why don't we give ourselves permission?

Try to feel your anger or grief as a process of grief-ing, of being in the grieving process as part of an ongoing effort that does not refer to the person or event that initially caused you to feel this emotion. As long as you attach a story to the emotion you will continue to feed your old belief systems and recurring programs in order to justify their self-righteous existence.

We live in a transformational time where commitment to our inner and outer truth alone will set us free. The New World can only be lived if we dare to change from within. It is therefore the full responsibility of the self to restore the light to the greater Self. Embarking on this invaluable personal work will serve us as individuals, but also the collective as a whole. We need the body, the instrument of the soul, to feel life. And only through the ability to feel can we transcend stagnated emotional blocks. It takes courage, and you can do it!

༄

In the beginning of this chapter, I shared my recent experience of walking through and meditating in a crop circle. This designated area, in the county of Wiltshire, England, embraces countless tiny farm villages in an agricultural eco-life. Again, the friendly nature of the people there, their faces radiant with love and joy, impressed me hugely. There was an energy that streamed directly from their hearts to touch my heart. Their willingness to step beyond the small self was palpable. It left me feeling humbled by the experience and reflecting on my personal life. Anybody who has ever had the chance to live among Tibetan natives knows what I am talking about. Their colored rosy cheeks, infectious smiles, and open hearts have an effect, solicited or not.

Living from the heart has an instant transference to anybody who comes in contact with this type of open energy. It is inevitable! When one person projects a heart-coherent field filled with care, love, and attention, all living organisms respond to the information in the field by becoming more receptive, soft, responsive, and connected to themselves.

When we are cared for or care for others, the heart releases a new pattern of information that deeply affects our physical make-up, especially our hormones and neurotransmitters. Then the brain follows suit.

It is my understanding that as the electromagnetic fields of the crop circles affect their surrounding inhabitants and the world, so do the inhabitants with their increasing energetic fields influence the quality and depth of the of the crop circle's formations and transmissions. The intricate designs of the crop circles display phenomenal patterns that offer to educate us on their spiritual and transformative messages—if we are willing to learn. Surely the creators have embedded timely technological instructions that could strengthen the survival of our planet! And since we know that electromagnetic fields react and respond to each other through resonating frequencies, we can only assume that their individual power and depth will increase.

I think it's safe to say that by now we fully recognize that the heart is much more than a pump! In doing so, we begin to understand how we, as a species, are intricately bathed and enveloped by shifting fields of heart-generated communication. Animals, plants, and humans are the colorful threads necessary for weaving this spectacular tapestry called the web of life.

We experience these communications not as lines of words on a page, but as multivalued, complex exchanges of intentionality, touches of the living intelligence of life forms to which we are kin. They are exchanges of qualities inherent in living organisms, not quantities of mechanical forces. We are one organism among many, one form among a multitude. —Stephen Harrod Buhner

A New World is birthed by deviating from the perception of the mind to the perception of living the path of the heart. One of the essential requirements for this spiritual transformation is to come to peace with pain. No expansion or evolution can take place without attention to the discomfort around change. Change involves challenging ourselves, an approach we so often perceive as a painful experience. Yet, becoming familiar with the pain is part of our growth and evolution. As we dare to walk to the core of the heart, our pain becomes more amplified, more uncomfortable. It can feel so unbearable and so challenging that we decide it's not worth it; that it's better to spend our entire life avoiding it. But the reality is that we are programmed to avoid the pain in order to separate ourselves from the soul. The joyful wedding with the soul requires this path of truth, as uncomfortable as the journey appears to be.

As we experience our world through our body, it is an indispensable companion. The body is not a separate thing, a living object, but a path we can take in getting to know the soul. We need the body to hear the soul! As we learn to know the soul, the body learns to experience life within as without. This is true for us personally and for the world. When the living body intertwines with the soul and the world, life becomes an embodied experience. At that point the marriage of the embodied soul and en-souled body is sealed.

The heart remembers this unity and in so doing remembers the unity and sanctity of the body. In this moment of remembering, we can touch and feel the beauty within. We feel softer, become more humble, and recognize that the consciousness of the heart is beauty itself. When the outer and inner worlds merge and unify, the idea of a duality between soul and body is foregone. To become an active participant in this New World requires action as well as active participation in experiencing the world through the heart.

Opening the heart requires the willingness to work with fear and love; both are required to find the authentic Self. It is easy to convince ourselves that closing the heart will keep us protected and safe. The surprise comes when we realize that courageously allowing the heart to stay open is what leads us to see that we have always been protected.

The human body is not an object in the world, but world as individuated consciousness. —Robert Sardello, Ph.D.

Are we prepared to take the risk to accept that illness and morbidity are essential companions on the path of healing and that planetary calamities are equally necessary to bring forth the awaited change? I ask you to consider that the capacity for change is embodied in each of us. It is what defines us—not our politicians, government, or institutionalized systems. Don't wait for the change to come to you: be the change. Your body is the junction between the visible and invisible worlds. When you let the two merge into one, pure energy will start flowing again. Once you learn to restore the flow, including those internal to the body, your physical being will be fully capable of restoring and repairing its "woundedness" by itself, and will naturally return to its state of dynamic balance.

Christianity's view that the body is a lower frequency and the soul a separate and higher frequency, not longer holds weight. A healthy and functioning body is not separate from a functioning soul, as they both belong to the same source field and are two faces of the same truth.

Core Soul

Inherent in all of us is the ability to heal ourselves through the influence of our highest intelligence. In fact, the sole purpose of the highest intelligence is to heal itself by healing the individual. When we observe flocks of birds in the sky or herds of deer turning and changing direction in total synchronicity we are witnessing coherent intelligence in action. Your soul carries the potential, as your mind carries the intention, as your brain produces the results, as your heart communicates with the brain and the world. We are living in an invisible field that somehow holds reality together, that somehow knows what is happening everywhere at once.

In *Quantum Healing* Deepak Chopra states: "The material body is a river of atoms, the mind is a river of thought and what holds them together is a river of intelligence. Every molecule in your body is wrapped up with a bit of invisible intelligence. If we want to navigate the field of intelligence, we must learn about it to the very depth, where the silent witness inside us awaits. To go deep means to contact the hidden blueprint of intelligence and change it."

By opening the heart in reverence and with a sense of wondrous awe, a feeling we may remember from childhood, we are able to receive the gifts of the soul. We already know the body is aware and highly intelligent. By tuning into the body, we not only increase its awareness but also clear the channel to the soul. Anytime we choose to grow and evolve we are tuning into the soul. As we continue the path in purifying our mental, emotional, and physical realms, we slowly start to integrate this daily requisite of living a soulful life. Only a balanced soul can influence the dis-eased body positively. When this happens the body has no choice but to shift and align with the soul's coherent frequency.

Allopathic medicine might call this event a remission of symptoms or an unexpected or "lucky" event for the patient. Yet, this healing is initiated by the alignment of similar, resonating frequencies manifested in complete recovery. The reason why not everyone manages to come to his or her full healing destiny might have more to do with circumstances or the ability to face a challenging path that often spans more than one lifetime.

Core Soul

Miraculous healing events have long been analyzed and deemed unexplainable. Such non-explanations might have been accepted in the past. But today and in the future the fundamental shift in consciousness will demand that we transcend this preconceived notion, as well as deviate from our excuses to avoid transformation. Today, our minds, bodies, and souls require the path of *Quantum Healing*, the path toward the deepest core of the mind-and-body system.

"When I'm ready," "This is too much for me," "I'm working on it," and "I can't deal with it now" are all self-generated excuses to embrace the patterns of the past, and will no longer be tolerated. The duo of the soul and the body is not prepared to accept this manipulative cowardice in the face of the individual and planetary emergent force that is carrying us with momentum and strength in a new direction. We are living in a time of diverse energy patterns, but cannot afford to live in the spaces between them. We need to make our decision! If we continue to resist the necessary steps to heal ourselves, we will only harm the body and avoid connection with the soul. The time has come to heed the call now, not tomorrow or in some future time or when you think you'll be "more ready" to leap.

Many of us have been noticing a strange sensation where time appears to be speeding up around us. It's as if we are losing control of something that was always absolutely dependable. This sensation feels puzzling and disconcerting. But I suggest it is a good thing! Dealing with an unsettling yet purposeful experience can catapult us back to the present moment. I hereby urge you to follow your emerging force asking you to live in the here and now.

In India, a rishi, or Hindu sage, experiences the changes of the world by acknowledging the changes within. External change is therefore a reflection of his or her change, and that change becomes a reflection of the change of the world. The individual's active participation is required and determines the outcome of the healing process or the choice to keep the war of duality alive within.

By becoming the observer the awakened mind is capable of choosing to be completely still, even in the midst of physical sensations, illness, thoughts, and emotions. From this seat of observation, we can

Core Soul

witness our experience even as we are experiencing that experience. Although you, the witness, silently stands in the eye of the storm, you are able to consciously dance with life at the same time, directly experiencing all sensations of the mind, body, and heart. Your consciousness, remaining grounded and still, dances with the experience.

Your dance is complete! From now on, life will become your eternal dance, easy and effortless. You have stepped beyond the veil of your own delusions and conditioned belief systems. You are free! Your dance is a reflection of your change, a testimony of your courageous and passionate intention to wildly move in the midst of stillness.

You don't have a soul.
You are Soul
You have a body.

—C. S. Lewis

Radical Dancing in a Soulful Place

Dancing is not rising to your feet painlessly, like a whirl of dust
blown about. Dancing is when you rise above both worlds,
tearing your heart to pieces and giving up your soul.

– Rumi

So many times throughout this book, you have heard me say that one's inner and outer environment influences cellular behavior, not only the genetic blueprint as believed by the more outdated approach. So far, the dance of healing has taken you far into the depth of your interior world of mind, body, and soul. You have bravely entered numerous unchartered territories within to discover the revelation of deeper layers waiting to be uncovered. This exciting dance will continue over the course of your life, as exploration is timeless and endless. Yet with each step your life is truly transforming into a magnificent piece of art. In this chapter, let's turn our attention toward our surroundings, to the chosen environments that consistently shape and color our lives.

Start by turning your eyes outward without letting go of your interior awareness and mindfulness. Let's explore the importance and value of your external energetic field, your place at work or home. Personally, beautiful, simple, life-affirming and sustainable environments always inspire my creative processes without diverting my attention from my exploration of self-growth.

Core Soul

External beauty feeds my soul, as my soul feeds on beauty; they go hand in hand, as they are partners.

Have you ever asked yourself which environment would suit you best? Are you thriving in a rural and green landscape or are you surviving in an inner city tower block? What do you need from your environment to truly heal? What does it take for you to create a harmonious place called "home"? Which environment gives you a sense of belonging? The radiance and resonance of your environment is equally important to the journey within, as they inspire each other.

Visit a quiet place. By now you know where to go. Close your eyes and envision the most nurturing and balanced place in yourself. See this place like a film passing in front of your eyes and enjoy its beauty, clarity, and radiance. Feel this place, see its colors, smell its fragrance, and look closely at the presenting details. What do you see? Are you looking at majestic mountains, the vastness of the blue ocean, or do you catch yourself listening to the soothing sound of flowing water? Feel your imaginary environment, its quality and its unique frequency. Then play your favorite music and start expressing this newfound vibration in your dance.

Dance and move like a mountain, defined and majestic, or as the ocean with its waves swaying back and forth without breaking its soothing rhythm. Dance and embody a small creek, skipping over small pebbles or perhaps dance out your city-fix. Whatever you require to thrive, express it in your dance. Then open your eyes and look around. Does your environment reflect your dance? Do you see anything around you, even if it is only a small object that mirrors your desired energy field? If you realize that your inner dream place, the place where you feel a true belonging, stands in total contrast to your external environment, then the time has come to initiate some changes in creating your true shelter of belonging.

Core Soul

Our environment influences our cellular behavior, as well as our relationship toward with ourselves. As we have entered one of the most important periods in human history with the opportunity to lift ourselves to a new level of consciousness that allows us to move toward healing, we are encouraged to radically participate in our environment with life-affirming and sustaining new ideas. Not only are we changing our position from experiencing life as a victim by becoming an active witness of our stagnated belief systems and suppressed emotions, but we are also becoming aware that we serve each other as mirrors of the soul. This concept can be confusing, as the form and quality of each individual path is completely unique to each of us. Don't expect everyone else to understand your journey. Especially if they've never had to walk your path. As we embrace both shadow and light, we dance the dance of love. In my experience, if a patient is set in motion, he or she will heal him or herself. This is the reason I believe in your dance!

Physical spaces contribute to the individual's identity and the way we respond and give back to our surroundings. Buildings and spaces hold memories of our personal experiences and can evoke in us a flood of physical sensations and emotions. A place takes on meaning as a result of stored sensations, often long upheld due to our attachment to them. We consciously avoid visiting certain places, as they remind us of old wounds and hurts powerful enough to stir up dormant feelings. As soon as we enter these energetic fields of the past, the heart remembers and registers this resonating frequency and responds to any related feelings. We might become emotional or melancholy or even begin to re-live the uncomfortable event internally. No matter if we are projecting our unresolved feelings onto a place or the place itself radiates its unresolved past, such as a land cradling the memory of a blood-drenched war that took place eons ago, we are affected by the interrelationship between our physical energetic field and the energetic field around us. Places that house such collective memories become dark and uninviting.

Core Soul

Across multiple environments, unhealthy ones are those that threaten safety by undermining the creation of social ties through abuse, violence, or conflict. A healthy environment, in contrast, provides safety, opportunities for social integration, and the ability to befriend all aspects of that environment.

Today, alarmingly, we have lost our sensitivity to places with a heart and soul. We choose our homes or apartments based on the spectacular view or convenience and amenity to the closest mode of transportation. We are more tantalized by contemporary design and futuristic architecture than the energetic field of the land or the home itself. Have you ever asked yourself: Who was this person who lived in my apartment before I moved in? What is the history of the land on which I built my house?

The constant change of managers at your local Italian restaurant might have little to do with the people themselves, but the unresolved history of the land on which the restaurant was built. Wherever there is a void of closure, the vibratory field lives on, particularly if it is negative and/or violent in nature.

So often we are unable to recognize the soul of a place due to our lack of cultural consciousness. When you connect with indigenous tribal cultures, however, the profound approach of sensing a place is still as common as the dawn greeting the sun. Here in the Southwest of North America, where much of the land is Native American, we are keenly aware of Gaia's moods and memories. Here, Nature is powerful and more unpredictable than we are, reminding us of the emotional field of Mother Earth. Ceremonies that include energy clearing, or "smudging" of polluted places with sacred sage and sweet grass, are as common as designing futuristic and sustainable living structures. This act of reverence and honoring the land pleases the Earth and makes her feel welcomed to the world of humankind. She loves being invited and will offer herself as a wonderful host at the same time.

Throughout time, we have progressively dulled our senses. Our natural antennas are less capable of feeling out our surroundings, which could inform us of nurturing or depleting natures that could affect our well-being. The control and love of power not only continues to dominate the planet, but also deeply penetrates our internal environment. Our hardened and impenetrable minds clearly reflect today's world, shaped by buildings made of indestructible concrete and unable to decay naturally. Many of us may have believed that increasing personal power would benefit the planet by making us all more powerful. But we do not all feel empowered. And energy that has been long suppressed will naturally find its way to the surface where it will burst like a volcanic eruption. As the female principle overtakes the old patriarchal paradigm, Earth is speaking out, letting us know that she too is changing. She doesn't want or need to be dominated anymore. Frankly, she has had enough. She wants to be heard, respected, and seen, as each one of us also desires.

The first step in sensing one's environment is waking up from the stupor of sensory numbness that seems to dominate our culture. Not only do we agree to suppress and deny emotional and physical pain, but we also seem to believe that it is acceptable for us to senselessly end the lives of other living organisms, including the planet itself. This is nothing but self-centered ignorance.

The soul does not reason and does not interpret, nor is it bound to any place. It is an energy filling a void in space. The journey of liberation and merging with the soul reveals itself as a continuous movement, an eternal dance, which by its nature has to move to transform. Your journey of healing is therefore an on-going process, which will expand over the course of this life and beyond. The journey of your healing has no beginning and no end; it is lived in the present moment, free of past and future references.

In my early years, I traveled a lot, and my excursions took me to the most amazing places. India, for example, is a country that certainly evoked all my senses. Being away from the familiarity of places and people, each and every day was filled with the unknown. Each day became a unique experience. As my mind stepped to the background, my senses came to the foreground as reigning and embodied internal guides. As my heart resonated with my surroundings, qualities of general criticism, cynicism, and judgment slowly fell away. If you travel to foreign countries, particularly alone, and especially as a woman, your senses need to operate at maximum capacity, directly informing you of the quality and integrity of places and people.

During the act of traveling we all strengthen our intuition. Intuition serves our survival, as it serves our creativity. This sense of knowing is a perception beyond all the physical senses and is meant to assist us on our journey.

Intuition is the wonderful moment when you pick up the phone knowing who will be at the other end before she says hello. It is the moment that effortlessly guided me to the appropriate references that I needed to write this book. It is the artist's strong conviction to paint his next painting with blues, not reds. Intuition serves our inspiration by stimulating our soulful creativity. Gary Zukav, author of *The Seat of The Soul*, describes intuition expressed through the higher Self as the connecting link, the language between the soul and the personality. The experience of having an intuition can't be explained in terms of the five senses, because it is the voice of our primal instinct that emerges from deep within. The time has come to reconnect and trust your core instincts, your intuitive knowing.

When we travel to foreign lands we become foreigners ourselves. Everything seems fresh, exciting, and full of new impressions. This is because we really don't know what will happen as each day unfolds unpredictably. During our travels, we feel free and unattached to the presenting events. We allow our mind to willingly serve the soul rather than control the part of us that perceives life as an ever-fresh experience.

Most of my life I lived in foreign countries, which meant learning new languages and adapting to new customs and codes of behavior. Although not always an easy path, I welcomed its newness and the potential for recreating myself.

Our attachment to places and objects defines our relationship to the present moment. It is almost impossible to stay in an objective mode relative to one's environment when we choose to feed a possessive and materialistic approach about external objects. This propensity for ownership is based on the same energy principle as the one that convinces us to act from our distorted personality rather than live from a place of emotional non-ownership, even with regard to our own soul.

Core Soul

The journey to find oneself belongs solely to the soul of the individual who mindfully witnesses the polarization between it and his personality. Being a traveler on the path of the soul's journey is always a singular one, even if we live and interact with each other. The witness's evolving awareness in combination with an externally harmonious environment can culminate in a passionately exhilarating meeting . . . a demanding, yet utterly rewarding process. They go together.

☙

Our home and personal space often puts forth the most resistance to change. Here, our memories and attachments have accumulated more than anywhere else. From clothes, furniture, books, and pictures to personal jewelry, this giant memory bank is fully stocked, sometimes with warm, family-orientated vibrations and sometimes with the most destructive and violent experiences. Your home defines your soul, as your soul defines your home.

Again, if we have rheumatoid arthritis and live in a damp abode, our arthritis is not likely to heal, no matter the medication we ingest. If we have a severe allergy to cat hair we will either have to treat it for considerable time—or find a new living arrangement for the cat. Whatever decision we make, we all have to respond to the situations that are presented to us. We do not have to wait until we experience physical symptoms that force us to look at our circumstances before we change our limiting environments.

Today, we are all asked to become active participants in our journey of self-discovery. We all want to live in a place called home, as we all yearn to live from an inner place called soul.

Anyone who is lucky enough to own a piece of property with land and gardens knows only too well how these invaluable green havens instill us with an undeniable emotional and physical well-being.

Whenever I feel out of balance, for whatever reason, a hike into the mountains, a walk through a botanical garden or my local park, or a stroll through the local garden center always does the trick. Here in the midst of Nature, even if it is man-made, my overactive nervous system immediately calms down and realigns itself. It is an instant remedy!

By now I hope we can all agree that the body isn't just a mechanical device and the soul isn't just an ethereal phenomenon, that both are interdependently related and that the existence of one is conditional on the existence of the other. Since the quality and resonance of one's inner and outer environment influences the manifestations of dreams and visions, to cultivate a beautiful thriving garden within requires an external environment that freely and without restriction supports this inner growth.

In a society based on excess productivity, corporate financial wealth, and personal power rather at the expense of authentic power, the importance of a sustainable and life-affirming environment is often seen as a diversion rather than a necessity. In the midst of amplified noise levels, radiation, and toxic pollution, however, the body and soul can hardly be heard or seen. Your demanding inner journey ideally requires a beautiful, purified, and calm external environment in order to be able to take these inner transformative leaps. The resonance of your environment therefore becomes an essential requisite for your personal evolution.

Allopathic medicine encourages this polarization in comparison to integrative medicine, which prefers to find new ways to merge all parts into a wholesome totality. Illness cannot be dissociated from the sick host, nor can the patient be detached from his mental and emotional imbalances. The presenting diseases of the 21st century will be more and more of a chronic nature, depleting vitality and productivity and consuming time and money. Heart diseases, diabetes, obesity, asthma, and depression are man-made creations, however, which can be moderated by how we design and build the human environment.

We shape our environment around us to achieve a particular function. Our homes should provide comfort, our workplaces should support productivity, and our hospitals should make us healthy. The choices we make in designing and operating these spaces are fundamental in achieving the desired outcome.

There is now widespread consensus that a hospital's physical and energetic environment has a direct effect on the patient's outcome and recovery time. Factors such as space, lighting, use of color, acoustics, noise levels, smells, and the degree of control a patient has over his immediate healing space all have an impact on the mood and overall well-being of the individual.

Research studies suggest that a noisy environment or artificial lighting can disrupt the brain development of premature babies. Alzheimer's patients exhibit less aggression, anxiety, and fewer psychotic symptoms when they are placed in private rooms with their own personal objects around them. A well-chosen healing environment not only enhances the patient's potential for full recovery, but also encourages his soul to participate in this challenging process. Hospitals that paint their cardiology department walls green have reported increased improvements in the symptoms of their patients. The physical heart responds well to the color green, which promotes the heart chakra of balance and love.

When we speak of health improvements we generally only focus on the most significant influences such as poor diet or the need for more exercise. If we were to direct our attention equally on potential health hazards, like the quality of housing, land-use, transportation, and architectural and urban design, we would consciously move toward the direction of planetary change. Why, then, does staying within the comfort zone seem more appealing?

If we only could accept the fundamental reality that the interdependence of our health and environment is an essential key in the maintenance of our individual and planetary health status, we might also awaken to the fact of the current collapse of our ecosystems and communities at large.

Studies show that children with asthma are particularly sensitive to air pollution. In the U.S. alone, 25% of children live in areas that regularly exceed the U.S. Environmental Protection Agency (EPA) limits for ozone, mostly due to car emissions. This staggering statistic can only be transformed when we start designing communities around people, rather than around automobiles. If we continue to resist these necessary changes, we will not only continue to burden the health of our children, but the health of future generations.

Over the past two centuries, the proportion of the world's population living in large towns or cities has grown from 5 to 50%—and is still growing. Urbanization has an enormous impact on our health, radically influencing cellular behavior. We can't pretend anymore that the global environmental toxicity, including radiation and climate change, does not characterize our lives today.

Numerous studies have shown that children have an increased susceptibility when exposed to toxicity, especially during their growth years when vital structures are developed and neurological connections established. During the first five years of a child's life, most of the development of the nervous system occurs, and yet we expose our children to a tsunami of chemicals which include mercury, lead, formaldehyde, and other carcinogenic substances, often disguised as binders and preservatives in vaccinations, as well as environmental, food-based, and household chemicals.

Giorgio Tamburlini, a doctor of pediatrics, epidemiology, and public health, states: "Since the nervous system has a limited capacity to repair any structural damage, if cells in the developing brain are destroyed by chemical such as lead or mercury, or if vital connections between nerve cells fail to form during critical periods of vulnerability, there is a high risk that the resulting dysfunction will be permanent and irreversible. The consequences can be loss of intelligence and alteration to normal behavior. Thus the fetus and infant have different vulnerabilities to damage than do adults and are in general more likely to suffer damage" (Rice and Barone, 2000).

Our children's metabolic pathways take at least six months after birth to become fully functional. It is evident that both prenatal and postnatal influences affect the newborn's neuroendocrine and neurotransmitter functions. It only makes sense that if the environment influences the physical functions of a newborn, it also influences all our daily interactions with each other and the world.

Pediatricians at the American Academy of Pediatrics have established links between pesticide exposure and a range of modern-day diseases in our children, from reduced birth weight and ADHD to impaired mental development. Mounting evidence suggests that increasing physical and mental health problems relate to human-modified places like homes, schools, workplaces, parks, industrial areas, farms, and roadways.

Core Soul

A health-supporting environment especially comforts people with mental health challenges. For many who are experiencing mental stress, commonly prescribed anti-depressants and tranquilizers often appear to be the only option. Today, new therapies like Ecotherapy emphasize the importance of physical activities like walking, gardening, and simply being in Nature for the depressed individual's state of mind. The needed change in us is clearly reflected by the needed change in our immediate environment. We are hereby encouraged in the participation in developing healthy and green spaces that promote community, including the provision for community-grown food, to improve mental, emotional, and physical health.

Our body and soul is like a divine garden, a living creation of abundance and growth. For a garden to thrive, it needs attention, love, and vital ingredients. A garden is also an empty space of non-judgment without attachment that allows us to relax and to deepen our connection to our Self. Your local park invites everybody, from lovers, to the homeless, to the office worker enjoying her lunch break. In the communal garden, we all have a bench and we all are invited.

Treat your body and soul like a communal garden. Allow all your organs and cells to rest in this place of rejuvenation and stillness. Such a divine garden can serve you by seeing and healing your soul. In this garden you can find a shelter of belonging, a sense of coming home, and peace. Your garden becomes your personal Garden of Eden. Once we understand the importance of living in and acting from our divine garden, embodied by the body and soul, we may feel more inclined to create external green gardens again.

Your environment reflects and influences the vibration, the quality, and the potentiality of your individual evolution, just as your body creates the needed terrain for your soul to heal.

༄

Look around your home, your workplace, your loft, your garage, the interior of your car, your closet ... the places you stuff with too many material items, most of which that are irrelevant to your life. Ask yourself: What do

Core Soul

I need in my life today? Do I really need this sweater I haven't worn for the last 10 years? Do I really need all these accumulated boxes of yard sale items piling up in my garage? Do I really need ten kitchen knives, although I mostly buy ready-made meals at the local supermarket?

May be it's time to de-clutter and organize your life as well as your environment in order to be able to tend your inner and outer garden. What you thought you needed five years ago may not be what you need today. Take some time to sort through all your cupboards, drawers, and personal items. Can you release yourself from some of these old attachments that hold you back in order to move on? Think about what is truly important in your life through the elimination of bad habits and the letting go of things that don't matter anymore. Be radical, be courageous, and let go!

Be your own interior designer. Create a fresh and joyful environment that stimulates all your senses. Cultivate a sense of wonder and innocence as you explore, like a traveler in an unknown country, your newly found terrain. The uncomfortable sensation of resisting the moment of letting go or the inner turbulence around indecision, confusion, attachment, and insecurity only hinder your ability to live with the flow. The release of old and lifeless items, as well as old stagnated belief systems, will heal you to your very core.

As you, the soaring eagle, look down and survey the entire personal landscape, evaluating, releasing, and eliminating your attachment to all, your future choices will birth a healthier and more sustainable inner and outer soulful garden.

❧

Your last dance, which will become your eternal dance, is imminent. I am pleased that you recognize the validity of a healthy environment for making inner changes and outer changes that mirror the change of this world.

I too decided to step out of my comfort zone, out of my well-defined, academic mental box. When I asked myself what

Core Soul

I really wanted to do, something radical and refreshing, something that would take me out of my current environment into a completely new environmental experience, the answer surprised me. I wanted to swim with wild dolphins! And this is exactly what I did. I booked a plane ticket to Hawaii with the intention of deepening my experience to live from my heart in a playful and joyful environment. The next chapter is infused with deep seawater wisdom, as my personal dance continued under the sea.

Dance, when you're broken open.
Dance, if you've torn the bandage off.
Dance in the middle of the fighting.
Dance in the blood.
Dance when you're perfectly free.

—Rumi

Your Eternal Dance Inspires and Transforms the New World

> Hidden beneath your feet is a luminous stage where you are meant to rehearse your eternal dance.
>
> —Hafiz

Beneath your feet indeed exists a world that invites you to participate in the unification of your soul and the soul of the world. The time has come to take the ultimate leap, not just for you, but also for the planet itself. There is no other way! How this event will look depends on your individual choices in setting your perfect stage for this transformative leap to occur. My path entailed swimming with wild dolphins in the Pacific Ocean along the Hawaiian coast.

The first excursion out, as I gently lowered myself from the boat with my fins, goggles, and snorkel into the cold vast ocean my nervous heart skipped a beat. Below me opened a nothingness of sheer blue space, embracing me with its giant arms. For a split second my mind created the worst scenario of the frightful image in being gobbled up by a shark only pushing my racing heartbeat further up into my brain. As I dared to look into the Big Blue below me, however, my heart softened. I became very still as I watched a pod of wild dolphins swimming right past me.

Core Soul

They were obviously enjoying themselves, swirling and twirling in the water and singing their song. A mother dolphin, turned on her back, supported her baby with her belly gently and with such care! These loving creatures not only looked after each other, but also exhibited their mindfulness with utter grace and beauty.

Deeply touched by this display of freedom, I too felt encouraged to finally let go of my fears and old belief systems. While I witnessed the surrender to the vastness of the ocean and myself, I instantaneously overflowed with a sweet sensation of love. The utter fear of a hypothetical death, as well as the fall of my splintered personality with its obsessive control mechanisms quietly slipped away in the face of this transformative event. In the presence of such magnitude we cannot help but crumble and feel humble. The idea of holding onto my fears clearly revealed itself as a self-destructive choice here that would only keep me from allowing myself to enjoy the present moment. The mental image based on a self-generated fear of a possible shark attack felt worse than letting go into the Big Blue. This is how the mind works at its worst and best.

Once I willingly dropped into my environment and the present moment by letting go of all mental analysis, I felt myself merging with the all-encompassing Oneness of my soul and the soul of the world. The dance of letting go changed from an initially fearful event into an exquisite moment in life. The merging with something bigger than I am, in this case the vast ocean, became the stage of my eternal dance. Once you truly let go of all of your preconceived ideas and conditioned perceptions of life—a very limited outlook indeed—you will be held and nurtured by love itself. Then your love merges with the loving soul of the world. Your healing is complete! You have reclaimed freedom of choice and authentic power to heal yourself and the world.

Core Soul

Dare to engage in something life-affirming that exists outside your known comfort zone, something outside and beyond your skin, something that pushes you courageously over your controlled edge. Then see and open your eyes! Your already-mastered dance will become spectacular.

The courageous act in stepping away from the ownership of one's conditioned ideas and preconceived perceptions not only initiates a profound transformative process for the individual, but also for his community, nation, and the planet. As you change, so will the world! Today, the ultimate shift in consciousness depends on the individual's infiltration and participation of the world with his new energy field. And, vice versa, the New World will respond by re-aligning and healing the cellular behavior of the individual.

Current catastrophes, from unprecedented massive oil spills to hurricanes and floods, political unrest to financial meltdowns, clearly remind us that we are all sitting in the same "evolutionary boat," no matter which part of the world we inhabit. This life-long, energetic marriage with our environment, based on symbiotic and sustainable relationships rather than separate dualities, creates a completely new and individualistic eternal dance. Your intention and subsequent decision to evolve instantaneously influences your close environment and then beyond. Your individual, evolutionary process influences humanity in its entirety, as well as planetary consciousness. This shift reflects a new level of understanding that all life is interconnected, interrelated, and interdependent.

During one of my dolphin swims, I noticed a baby dolphin dragging a long fishing line from its tail that had to be at least 100 feet. I knew the baby would die unless it was soon freed from its man-made instrument of torture. Seeing such unnecessary and upsetting scenes should serve to remind us that we live in a very fragile and interdependent ecosystem, one meant to enrich all living organisms. Luckily this sad event came to a happy ending. One of the crew members dived into the ocean's depth and released the dolphin baby from its tether. Once you enter the animal or plant kingdom on this level, it is impossible not to appreciate the interrelationships and codependences that exist in this intelligent and ordered ecosystem. This example of humankind's aquatic pollution is another demonstration of humanity's utter deviation from wholeness. Delicate and overstressed ecosystems worldwide are seeing the effects from garbage, oil spills, and inhuman means to achieve need-driven ends. The ripples of devastation are certain to be felt for many generations to come, if not forever. Every human action against the environment, however, is an action against our own health and well-being. As the oceans and rivers—the bloodlines of Mother Earth—are filled with ever-mounting levels of toxic waste, so are our narrowed and blocked blood vessels filled with accumulating metabolic waste, plaque, and incoming environmental toxic chemicals. The state of our planet clearly reflects the state of the body and vice versa.

If we wish the world to make the shift toward a more peaceful and sustainable outlook long term, we have to first start with ourselves. As we enter the era of conscious evolution, we come to understand that love alone is not enough anymore. The New World demands responsible choices and mindfulness combined with a consistent and active participation along with love if we expect to see a brighter future. As long as we continue to operate from the platform of personal gratification and selfish motivations we only harm ourselves and the very nature of our existence. If we wish to see a world free of destruction, war, and hate, we will have to let go of fear.

Only through seeing and feeling our fears will we come to know that they don't belong to us. Our fears are our teachers; through them we come to know our worth, our path, and ourselves. The exposure of fear can only bring self-knowledge, freedom of choice, and ultimate healing. The choices that one makes in facing the fears will determine one's character and perception of life. One's character determines one's destiny: you are the author of your own story. Each and every challenging, if fleeting, situation we face is designed to push us into a quest for the deeper meaning, purpose, and intelligence resting behind them. As we consciously abandon and release our fears and tendency for criticism and judgment the larger planetary energetic field will do the same, this time in a positive example of cause and effect.

Ask yourself: *What are you really afraid of? What limits you in your life? What controls you?* For most of us, the answers are easy: your thoughts, your fears, and your beliefs, all of which shape and influence your personal perception of your environment and yourself.

Our planet currently offers us the opportunity to release our worn-out, unsustainable patterns. It is not enough anymore to consider letting go of our personal shadows or to contemplate undertaking personal future changes while prolonging the continuation of uncomfortable events and our engagement in them. From now on, recognize that the sole purpose of every encounter and circumstance serves you directly in your soul's need to heal and to merge with your Self, the planet, and the whole. Only by experiencing life in its totality will you set yourself free.

When we understand that we all come from the same creative pool and source, our outlook and general perception to life and the world will change. This new way of living requires the ability to use the senses with awareness and attention. Through this process of conscious feeling and sensing the environment and circumstances, our physical and spiritual heart will open like the petals of the most fragrant flowers. Then the heart's magnetic energy field will expand and reach far beyond the physical boundary or skin to touch the planetary magnetic energetic matrix. When we truly start to understand how we are all connected and dependent on each other, we will enter the realm of reverence and love. When the vibration of love enters our cells and heart, we will live and express beauty and joy.

Then, we will embody the soul! An authentically empowered person chooses to live in and through love. From this place any actions birthed from the splintered personality reveal themselves as meaningless endeavors and deviations from source. This is the reason why responsible choices are so important. When we limit the frequency of love to "romance" or squeeze it into a personal container through our definition, we are still acting and feeling from the place of the personality; we are trying to own and control this life-giving radiance. But love is an active phenomenon, a frequency that is the result of a shift in consciousness. Love freely arises from the heart as soon as we choose to participate in the larger picture. Love cannot be owned, as love owns us. Love is the image of the soul.

Core Soul

Lennon beautifully describes this idea: "There are two basic motivating forces: fear and love. When we are afraid, we pull back from life. When we are in love, we open to all that life has to offer with passion, excitement, and acceptance. We need to learn to love ourselves first, in all our glory and our imperfections. If we cannot love ourselves, we cannot fully open to our ability to love others or our potential to create. Evolution and all hopes for a better world rest in the fearlessness and open-hearted vision of people who embrace life."

Swimming with wild dolphins opened my heart in a sacred rite of passage, an initiation. Whenever I heard their happy song below my feet, I sang back to them, my heart melting and my tears of joy and laughter joining the ocean's fluids. When life begins to reflect such wonder and beauty, we allow ourselves to be deeply touched by love itself. At this point, the personality retreats into the background to willingly serve the higher purpose of the soul's assignment. Experiencing one's pure existence as unfolding creative energy transforms the initial paradigm of polarization where the personality and soul are splintered into a paradigm of endless learning to understand our rightful place in those terms. In order to heal and merge with the soul, we need to diverge from the path of duality and separation and choose the exquisite and sometimes complex path of unity common to us all. The many examples of how far we have deviated from our individual soulful unions are apparent in the depth and breadth of our physical and emotional disease. A wholesome life must entail the death of the ego and the health of the body.

Exploring the soul's path has led me to recognize that we already know how to find ourselves. Unfortunately, we have spent a long time numbing our sensory faculties and appear to have forgotten how to rekindle their flames. We can remember! You can ignite the flame of self-awareness by consciously setting the intention to walk the path of your liberation, by stepping out of or moving beside your meaningless mind chatter. By choosing not to engage in the daily mental entertainment, you may be surprised how nurturing life can suddenly be, despite its challenges. Only through the unfiltered perception of life can we experience the pulsing current of being alive. This requires that we stop talking and thinking so much and start mindfully observing the world without our personal filters of perception.

Swimming with wild dolphins in the ocean is one way to reduce all external audio distractions, as one can only hear and perceive one's own heartbeat and each silent breath going in and out. Anything else becomes irrelevant. Destructive thoughts and even heightened excitement instantly impacts the rhythm of the heartbeat and therefore the quality of breath. Being kissed by the face of the ocean is an experience that doesn't allow the mind to wander, as wandering instantly interrupts rhythmic and regular breathing via the snorkel and results in the rude awakening of swallowing way too much seawater.

As I focused on calming my mind and on the present moment, not only could I thoroughly enjoy myself, but found I was able to swim with the dolphins for a much longer period of time. This exercise clearly demonstrated to me how easily it is to be swayed by our mental distractions, to drown in these distractions . . . to drown in our own thoughts. Try to stay as open and present as possible in all your experiences. Do not attempt to influence the outcome or your expectations. Then your unfiltered perception will allow you to see reality as it is, rather than what you hope or expect to see.

Under the water, whenever I drifted outside my present awareness, I pressed all the fingertips of one hand into my sternum, located between the chest and the seat of the spiritual heart. As soon as I felt that external pressure going inward, my mind and breathing softened and relaxed, allowing me to re-center myself in the momentary activity again. I still continue to use this technique today. It works each and every time!

All animals, especially wild dolphins, resonate to this calm frequency by responding with their joyful and happy play. Their excited chin slapping on the water's surface or their engaging bow-waves as they ride alongside the boat signals approval of and invitation to us humans. Conversely, dolphins shy away from any aggressive behavior and negativity, frequencies that do not resonate with and are alien to their DNA. The cellular behavior of the dolphin responds to peace, play, and joy; this is as simple as it gets. When they are in their element they transfer this frequency to us. At its best it reminds me of watching happy children at play. We can all recognize this feeling, either by tracing back through the memory banks of our childhood or observing children whose play is timeless and pure in the here and now. Dolphins awaken the inner child within us with their carefree, blissful, playful side. Dolphins are a perfect example from Nature of how we should and can be.

Symbolically, dolphins often refer to playfulness, transcendence, gentleness, harmony, intelligence, contentment, creative self-expression, friendship, and generosity, as well as the connection to Self and power. In Christianity, the dolphin was portrayed as an aspect of Christ, a symbol of resurrection and the message of well-being to the pure-hearted. In Greek mythology, the dolphin was responsible for carrying the souls of the dead to the island of the Blessed. The dolphin was a companion of the sun god Apollo, representing life, activity, vibrancy, health, renewal, and intelligence, and to the moon goddess Aphrodite, with her qualities of hidden power, intuition, dreams, conception, and the feminine principle.

There are many reasons why dolphins are important in this context of healing and health. Primarily, though, the dolphin is connected to the principle of duality. As it is both mammal and fish, it exists in both worlds at once. Hence, another lesson we can learn from the dolphins is to view the marriage of our initially dualistic properties, represented by our splintered personality and soul, as an opportunity to live in both realms by viewing and engaging with life from an impersonal and neutral seat. To operate solely from a place of self-interested ego, to act only from the position of the soul to the point of being blinded, or to ignore the validity of this marriage altogether creates the ever-present and on-going imbalance within. Neither side can be ignored nor denied, as both aspects serve each other and reflect two sides of the same concept. The art of living from a neutral position requires the art of acknowledging both polarities.

Why not let allow a little chaos in your life from time to time and be glad for the unexpected? Why not seek the unusual and innovative? There is more to life than order, normality, and monotony. When life feels static and without a natural sense of flow, open yourself to the opportunity for change and upheaval, as it might bring new beginnings and a fresh perspective.

꙳

If you ever have the chance to swim with wild dolphins, you will notice how they protect each other and look after each other, and also how they act the same way in their interactions with humans. Dolphins are sociable mammals; to see a dolphin by itself would be in opposition to its nature. Dolphin communities stay together, though immediate families often split off from time to time in smaller units. Highly intelligent, they take care of other injured or needy animals, acting with care and compassion. They have been known to bring incapacitated or distressed members of their group to the surface of the water to help them breathe the life-saving air. These acts of caring kindness, called epimeletic behaviors, have been extended to humans as well, where the dolphins have helped lost or stranded individuals find their way back to shore or have kept them above the surface of the ocean until help arrived.

The spirit of the dolphin is generous and knows no boundaries. Dolphins willingly take on the role of "watchers of the waters." How about if we as a conscious and awakened species step up to the plate and become watchers of our individual and planetary souls? A very new concept indeed! Our evolutionary consciousness today requires that we open ourselves unconditionally, as the dolphins do, and recognize the great gift they give us in awakening us to a higher frequency on our journey to wholeness.

Somehow we have forgotten about this natural receptivity in our focus on shifting our priorities to the mind, a faculty that naturally chooses movement and stimulation. But behind the need to keep the mind chattering lies the need to protect and defend at all cost. Constant analysis and intellectualization in the present moment may seem to create a feeling of power and control for the one who rejects and fights a larger perspective. But this kind of protection is false. It satisfies only momentarily, as the ego can never be content. Inner growth can only be achieved if you yield this seat of personal power. To find peace and contentment requires selfless surrender to your deepest Self.

Core Soul

By observing and witnessing the voice of that part of yourself that needs to know and control, you set the decision to move into a different and higher frequency of life. If used with mindfulness and intention, your mental chatter and tyrannical attitude can become the launching ground for true spiritual awakening. When you get to know the one who watches the neurosis within, you will get to know a very different you. By stepping back from the personality and becoming the witness to the thoughts and feelings, you will become part of the world's energy field, a shift that allows you to see and live a new reality. Then, you truly experience who is experiencing the experience!

Allow yourself to see that your present circumstances don't determine your destination, but serve you as pointers in your responsible choices to come. It is the nature of the false personality to never be content or quiet; this attribute doesn't belong to its nature. But there is no need to change it in its form or core. It is as it is. It is an essential part of your make-up and rightfully deserves its existence along with all the other parts of you.

※

In the beginning of this book, I shared my near-death experience of almost drowning in a lake. But I only recall this event fondly. Why? Because from the perspective of a small child the sense of merging with the water's depths in all its exquisite stillness was far from traumatic. I was not thinking, but using all my senses. Rationality had no place in my experience. I saw the world through the eyes of a child, and not through an adult's more "rational" vision. Falling into the water was an experience involving every sense, of touching, seeing, hearing, tasting, and even smell, bypassing the all intellectualized exploration. In that instant, I was the water, and I was the stillness at the same time. In that moment, I went beyond myself to allow the realm of senses and no limitations. There was no fear!

Half a life span later, faced with a similar moment, I realized that I was reacting with my adult "rational" mind. In doing so, the experience could easily become a nightmare if I let myself be taken over by my hypothetical fears. What kept me from traveling down that path was recalling my former, completely different and magnificent experience as a child. Although my mind was choosing to fuel the sensation of terror instead of choosing to experience the ability to float in clear, safe water, my willingness to step into consciousness transformed my fear into expansiveness similar to that which I'd felt in the lake as a child.

To go beyond fear requires courage at the core of our being. Taking those initial steps might require all that we've got. We might feel pushed against the wall or leveled to the ground until we feel ready to surrender to something bigger than ourselves. This is the same predicament that rules humanity today. Growing into the Self means that we no longer have to go to such extremes in order to wake up. We can stop holding on to one or the other—the dark or the light side of our Self—and be one with both. As judgment fades, the smaller self, based on duality, retreats into the background, opening the doors to an all-encompassing and soulful life.

Floating on the face of the Pacific Ocean taught me well how to witness my fears and step behind them in order to expand my inner and outer vision. Once I tasted the quality of being the one who witnesses, the one in me who isn't afraid of my mind and thoughts, the one who decides to jump beyond hurdles and willingly leaps into freedom, I could not only hear the beat of my heart, but the beat of my soul. Then the path of freeing myself became as luminous as Mother of Pearl.

༄

Your first leap may be the most frightening one, yet I can reassure you that each one that follows gets easier and more exciting. Evolution is a series of breakthroughs and often occurs at that point when we know our only option is to give up. Any breakthrough at the level of the soul brings us closer to love, but also to its challenges. Try to see every step as part of the process. Actions and thoughts birthed from a place of consciousness resonate a quality of pureness and clarity and confirm the ever-deepening path of truth. Everything else non-constructive in nature falls away in time, as you will have no interest in inviting such deep negativity anymore At this point, you can begin to peacefully observe your immediate natural environment, as well as the nature of your individual expressions. From that moment, life becomes easier and simpler on all levels.

With this approach to life, you are sure to find that many things in your environment will change—relationships, jobs, health issues, and your relationship to spirit itself. You will experience life as it happens by witnessing it all! You then start accepting what is, rather than feeling like a victim of what is happening to you. I am not postulating that life will be a rosy ride from now on, but I can share with you that from that moment on you will be far less occupied by the relentless fears and desires that keep you from seeing the reality of the presenting life experiences. Whether you are dealing with environmental catastrophe or deep personal loss, you will be reminded that you are walking the chosen path of living awareness. Ask yourself: *Do I want to live a life-affirming and health-promoting life? Do I want to be happy? Do I see my life from the posture of a victim by continuing to struggle and blame my environment?*

In my experience, stress only occurs when I resist life's events. By witnessing any event in its totality, without ignoring it or feeling attracted to it, I can simply be present. As I express a peaceful state of being, peace enters my life. From this seat of neutrality, even physical pain or debilitating illness cannot yank you out of your place of serenity. It simply cannot, as the personal game is over. You might feel the sensation of pain, but as you do not personalize your pain anymore it becomes a fleeting sensation traveling in and out of your consciousness. In our language, we refer to this form of existence as an awakened state or enlightenment, but such words were and are still reserved for chosen souls in religious and spiritual circles. That's why I simply call it "free to be." It is easier to relate to this journey as a simple endeavor, rather than something unattainable or a privilege for religious and spiritual leaders. This journey belongs to us all, to men and women, to all other living organisms, and to the planet. This journey should be free of tension and constriction, as it serves to encourage you to go a step farther and to leap a little more every day.

Core Soul

In the brilliant words of John O'Donohue's Anam Cara: "Once the soul awakens, the search begins and you can never go back. From then on, you are inflamed with a special longing that will never again let you linger in the lowlands of complacency and partial fulfillment. The eternal makes you urgent. You are loath to let compromise or the threat of danger hold you back from striving toward the summit of fulfillment."

Along with this kind of new perception may come the feeling that you're missing some spice in your life as its familiar mental and emotional drama has been erased. Suddenly life becomes more of a neutral experience, rather than one filled with the daily turmoil of ups and downs. This new energetic environment requires some adaptation, not only for the one who experiences it, but also for his mind and body. In this new field of relating to one's Self, life's old paradigms and patterns will be exchanged for a clear and pure perception infused with awareness, the essence of consciousness. It is like re-booting an outdated computer after it has been upgraded with brand new technology and possibilities. As life and the world cease to be a problem, this experience of neutrality will become an exquisite requisite for living a joyful and soulful path fueled from your very core.

As you experience and perceive life from an impersonal position, the seat of your consciousness, difficult situations and destructive thought patterns hardly faze you anymore. If you catch yourself being impulsive or reacting to a disturbing situation or person, you now have the tools to snap yourself out of it in a much quicker and constructive way. As time unfolds, you become stronger and more confident in choosing a tremendously expansive life compared to the current limited, false one. From now on, this new unfolding frequency will continue to sustain you through all your life. Rather than looking for the answers outside you, you are the answer... and always have been.

The commitment to make the leap to choose freedom and to liberate the part of you that has been waiting for you all along will change your life. As soon as we stop entertaining the melodrama, our spiritual path has begun. To be free isn't only determined by countless meditation practices, the next best physical exercise, or the newest diet plan, all of which appear to do the work for you. The first leap starts with you and your intention, devotion, and commitment to unite with your soulful being. The effects of this fundamental and profound choice are and will be life-changing. Recognize the awesome power of choice here! The trillions of cells in your body will rejoice that moment of bold decision, as your body will finally have been given the space to heal and your cells will finally be able to awaken to the code of self-liberation embedded in the soul. Choose awareness over personal control and suffering and your profound healing will fall naturally into place.

There is a reason why we hold onto our thought patterns. After all, they are familiar and tangible. But stepping beyond the irrational fears and personal desires opens up a vast void, one predictably less tangible and certainly without an instruction manual. Due to its unfamiliar and more etheric nature, we may choose to stay closer to the splintered and battered personality than take what seems like a risk to live from the spaciousness of the soul. The personality is predictable and controlled, while the soul is unpredictable and spontaneous. Yet as we scramble for certainty in the face of our eternal dance, we ultimately sacrifice more and more solid ground in our need for safety.

As we are all part of a much bigger and dynamic evolutionary process, our souls and the soul of the world are dancing together in constant flow. The mind may feel as if it is vaulting into an endless void, but the heart feels as if it is coming home. It is that easy, and it doesn't require any religion or special spiritual path. It does not need a label, as it has always been our true core existence all along. Being awake and consciously participatory in this New World isn't something we have to name, nor do we have to consider it "special" in any way. The time has come to live from this new perspective and approach your relationship to life and the world as you would your need to eat and drink every day . . . as a basic fact of life. Give yourself permission to sense and experience life, rather than relate to it from a personalized controlled posture. Your body will instantly respond to this change.

The act of allowing life to be experienced, of witnessing and learning from whatever we come in contact with, encourages the physical cells of the body to let life pass through, rather than interfere with their natural flow. The circulatory system, from the blood to the lymph, will flow in a harmonious, unobstructed manner rather than be pushed to overcome blockages or constrictions. When the cells are able to communicate with each other again they can support the process of overcoming physical emergencies and illness, in the same way that the dolphins support each other by bringing the distressed animal or person to the water's surface. With this newfound constructive dialog the body is given new life and all cells are provided with an energetic healthy environment in which to live. Such an environment will positively influence their behavior and proliferation now and in the future.

What we do to our planet will never stop having an impact. Neither will what we do to the body. Even more importantly, since there is no real difference between the two, what is happening outside of us is a reflection of what is happening inside. Resisting or allowing movement in life is what makes or breaks the quality of our existence. Remember, congestion creates disease just as circulation creates health. Let your dance be the flow!

ಊ

To live from a place of presence and awareness doesn't mean operating from a place of stagnancy or non-movement. Our true center, called source, is never stagnant, never balanced, but in a constant state of harmony in motion. Imagine floating in the middle of the river and letting yourself be carried by the water without resisting its flow. If you attempt to resist the flow, to go upstream or force your way to shore, you are fighting the natural course. In the body such resistance interferes with its natural rhythm and desire to stay in motion. The condition of optimal health requires being and living the movement of each and every day. To speak of a balanced universe would be to speak of a stagnant and non-alive experience of being alive. Being alive means living in peace in the middle of the hurricane all the time!

Spiritual evolution is about experiencing life rather than making it. Even as a child, I somehow knew that this was the way to live a meaningful versus an enslaved life. When you follow the movement of experiencing life, you listen more carefully to your body's requirements. It will tell you when it is hungry, when it needs a rest, or when it needs to replenish its energy. It will tell you when it needs help and when it is able to meet an emergency by itself. It will also tell you when it needs you. The art of communication between you and your body will become an essential part of your future well-being. Again, here too, I learned so much from my friends the dolphins.

Humankind has long been intrigued by the idea of communicating with other forms of intelligence outside our human form, from the apes, elephants, dolphins, and whales to extra-terrestrial life forms. Dolphins communicate almost solely by sonic transmission, using sonic and ultrasonic waves to scan their surroundings by identifying objects by shape and distance. The most astounding fact is that dolphins perceive incoming information as aural or holographic input, which requires no translation through any other medium in order to be communicated. Their communication is efficient and much more accurate than our own, as less information is lost in the process. The informative input is immediate, direct, and precise.

Imagine if we could communicate with each other without verbal misunderstanding and without needing so many contexts. Would not the world be a better place? I believe a greater degree of intimacy would develop and result in fewer personal and global wars and greater, more beneficial exchanges. We recognize such moments when we deeply connect with a loved one without verbal communication, when our minds seem to be joined and words are unnecessary. Communicating with the environment and with Self can be the same way, feeling the direct transmission of clear incoming messages regarding our next steps and direction. These rare moments of powerful intimacy with your Self, your body, and your environment should now become the norm, not the exception, as you dance into a very different way of living.

The dolphin's echolocation language is critical to their survival and very essence. Not only does it serve as a means for locating food and detecting predators, but as a means for the deepest kind of bonding. Humans could learn a great lesson from these creatures by practicing how to invoke the natural senses in a new kind of communication.

Core Soul

The fact is that we too are able to transmit and receive information in an unfiltered and clear way. The first step is to cultivate that conversation with your body, your organs, and your cells. Tune into each part and let it speak to you. Let the conversation begin and see how intimate your relationship to your body can be ... like two souls joined without speaking a word. Soon you will notice that your aural field has begun to expand and exceed your physical boundaries to include direct communication with the environment as well. This new way of communicating with your body is the link to unambiguous and unequivocal communication with your soul.

Dolphins not only teach us to communicate in a new and effective way with each other, but inspire us to develop a new method of understanding, experiencing, and interacting with the environment. Their joyful resonance streams through us and activates the realm of our heart. During this transfer of information, not only do we feel more deeply, but simultaneously activate and re-kindle any dormant memory banks in our body and cells. The dolphin's presence reminds us to feel our true selves, an essential requisite for this new way of living.

As we deepen the communication within with our thoughts, emotions, and physical cells, we enhance and amplify our inherent cellular intelligence and general receptivity to healing. Trillions of cells are now ready to communicate and work with each other, rather than operate from the principle of hierarchy and personal power. We must understand that actively participating in our core healing takes place via the feelings, not solely through changes in the body's vibrational frequency. When we do, we realize the responsibility inherent in the quality of our thoughts and feelings. We may have a lot to adjust to and re-learn in order to become an instrumental part of this New World, yet every little effort is actually required. This new method of communication is available to everyone and only requires you to make it happen, to absorb it permanently into your cells.

As we enter the age of soul-consciousness, we will have to give birth to our own essence. Such an event comes with this new uncharted territory. At this stage of human and planetary evolution, we are encouraged to contemplate the basic fact that we do not live only for or within ourselves anymore. The re-building and re-organization of a self-sustainable planet necessitates a continual, ever-changing relationship between our souls and the soul of the world.

We all recognize the beauty of a dynamic and vital relationship between two lovers, which demonstrates its individual character in its fluidity and movement. The dance between two lovers is fresh, spontaneous, and playful. Yet, if this dance of unhindered frequencies comes to a halt the relationship between the lovers soon deteriorates in the way a lifeless body appears drained of its blood.

The individual's relationship to the environment determines the ultimate dance with the unknown, the unpredictable, and innovative. Each step is unique; each twirl unfolds from the place of originality and spontaneity; each sound can only be heard once. No move has ever been practiced, known, or seen before.

Living this way requires the development of our given senses in the way the dolphins sense the environment and the planet. To actively participate in positive change requires that we fine-tune our sensory capacities to establish an aural communication field, like listening without hearing actual words. It requires us to touch without actually touching, to taste without the actual need to chew, to smell without the need to follow the trail of fragrance, and to see with our inner vision rather than our eyes. Once the senses are fully activated and integrated as essential tools for perceiving incoming information, we will be able to hear, touch, taste, smell, and see love again. Love is the essence of the soul and serves the essential purpose of bringing us closer to ourselves. Feel the world instead of trying to understand it. Follow the impulse of your soul.

We cannot deny the fact that the time has come to get in touch with our feelings, the feminine aspect of natural law and nature. As the paradigm of duality comes to a close, we recognize that the soul of the world, a living being, lives both inside and outside of us. This new purpose and meaning of life requires us to learn how to love and honor ourselves as the other.

This time of purification and preparation for living a new dimension entails the death of the limited individual and the death of the personality. This also means that we are entering a new era of stepping beyond personal love into the experience of unconditional love by acknowledging the soul of something bigger than us. You might say we are graduating from our personal love into an all-encompassing spiritual love by living from the consciousness of the heart rather than the mind. As a new kind of love emerges from within, so emerges a new kind of spiritual humanity. The merging of the individual soul with the soul of the world will connect families, communities, nations, and the planet as a whole. This may sound far out for some of you, but the signs are already here to verify this planetary movement.

To fully manifest this process, which has already begun, we are called to wake up from the sleep of thinking we are defined and programmed, when we do not need to be. Taking this fundamental step of ultimate personal healing, we will change the world so much in need of healing. When you wake up to your own magnificence and authentic power, as well as to your truth, you will also sense peace and love. It is inevitable. Then you will see the uniqueness and magnificence in everyone and everything else around you.

Humanity is now experiencing a new sense of love. We are not carried by this love, nor do we fall into it! This love originates in us. We create love by waking up to ourselves! This doesn't mean the personal romantic notion of love has to be left behind. On the contrary, our personal relationships will be stabilized and strengthened in a way that will contribute to the birth of the more self-empowering, spiritual aspects between two partners, whether in love or business.

༄

Throughout this book, we have explored the path of freeing the individual soul by stepping away from the splintered personality. Let's take it a step further! Now the individual soul, already in place, needs to free itself from its individuality in order to merge with its outer world through its senses. At this point you are not only healing yourself, but also participating in the healing of your personal and greater natural environment.

With this new sense of love we will be able to see and relate to individuals and nations in their totality and as a unified entity. Here, the idea of you and I as separate beings only results in the same false assumptions of the past. The individuality we once cherished and defended now belongs to the world. To fully express this vision we are asked to transform from within.

This New World is ready to open her heart and soul to a society that is unashamed to welcome her as a living entity and a representative of the female principle. This is not a new concept; in fact it is thousands of years old, as all indigenous cultures honor the inherent female qualities in all Earth-bound natural laws. To them, the reverence of Mother Earth comes as easily as the sun rises each day.

Robert Sardello, in *Love and the Soul*, comments: "The new soul practice means to expand our experience of the ego to the point that the sense of who we are incorporates all of the world, which at the same time means that where we find our individual soul is in all of the world."

Being a witness to the dolphin's unconditional love toward its own kind and to humans demonstrates its selfless role in inspiring the development of our present consciousness. Living a life with mindfulness and awareness is the result of living from the heart rather than the analytical mind alone.

The society we have known is rapidly changing from one with a consciousness based on self-gratification to one with a more heart-centered consciousness. In order for this to happen we have to go along with the change as opposed to fear it. The process of great global and personal transition has begun. Any effort to resist this natural emerging force will only prolong the inevitable.

The New World seeks an embodied love, a love that can be found within and without the codependency on the environment. By listening to the teachings of your soul you will find love, embodied in us all. This journey of the soul invites us to join a society whose consciousness is based on the individual as well as the whole. Raising a consciousness fueled with the understanding of a heart-bound society is not a small change—a general shift toward a better humanity—but a fundamentally different way of relating to each other. It is indeed a New World! Opening up to our emotional realms should not be such a frightening or terror-inducing endeavor anymore, as more and more value is placed on the depth and breadth of our feelings in sensing the world around us. Emotional healing is therefore the next phase of the journey. To live a spiritual life doesn't imply an out-of-body experience, but full participation with the body and soul. To live, think, feel, and act from the heart will dissolve the separation between the world and its living organisms. We are entering the era of becoming whole, not just ourselves, but also all humanity. If we continue to turn away from the world as a totality, we will continue to turn away from the body, too. Clearly, without this fundamental paradigm shift in consciousness, the future of humanity is at risk.

As Rudolph Steiner suggests: "Love must turn to the self, only in order to turn self into service in the world; the rose adorns herself only in order to adorn the garden."

In this New World your decisions and responsible choices not only belong to you, but are also an expression of the Earth's consciousness. Whatever you strive for or set in motion has to be seen in the context of the whole, with an understanding that favors the Earth-body connection.

As the circulating blood is an aspect of the body's participation, so are thoughts and actions, which directly influence the totality of a healthy world. The body houses about 70 to 100 trillion individual cells, which interact with each other each and every second with elegance, intelligence, and kindness. Surely, it must be possible to create a sustainable and healthy system for the nearly 7 billion people on this planet, a tiny fraction of the job that the body has to perform on a daily basis. To live from wholeness by creating an integrated expression that ultimately serves the totality of humanity in the same way our physical cells serve the totality of the living body is not just a dreamy ideology or some new-age idea, but one that belongs to reality. This proven and well-established concept is happening in your body while you are reading this book.

As the mind shapes the character of the cellular community, so do governments in relation to their citizens. The principle and its nature are the same, as both aspects can only begin to thrive with an understanding of their interrelationship and interdependency. You only have to look at the most creative and intelligent life-giving mechanisms within your body to understand the requirements and inherent laws of creating an outer self-sustainable and healthy world.

We really do not need to invent new strategies or concepts. All we need is the humility to look within and the answers will be given, right here and now. It might not seem evident to us now, but the future of our species and the planet truly lies in our hands and within the present consciousness. We are able to rewrite our own stories, just as we are able to use all our life experiences as teachers and lessons serving the unfolding evolution. The power to change is within us!

Both individual work and planetary participation will be based on our being integral participants in and observers of life at the same time. This dual-sensory faculty, an essential requisite in the New World, therefore requires an inherent and alive sense of awareness.

≈

My experience with wild dolphins already had exceeded my expectations, but a final observation regarding their sleep patterns led me to even deeper understanding.

Whales and dolphins are mammals and in lot of ways just like human beings. They have a similar bone structure, are warm-blooded, and give birth to living young. Of course, the biggest difference lies in the fact that they live in the water and we on land, which speaks to their very different breathing mechanism. Human beings and other mammals breathe with their lungs involuntarily, meaning our breathing happens on its own accord. Whales and dolphins, on the other hand, have a unique respiratory system that allows them to be under water for some time without breathing in any oxygen. But remember, breathing with their lungs the way we do still requires that they come up to the water's surface to get their needed oxygen. This phenomenon makes them "conscious breathers," actively having to decide when to take the necessary breath, or suffocate instead. Consequently, in order to breathe, dolphins and whales must be conscious. So, what do they do when they need to rest or want to sleep? The answer is one of Nature's most intelligent and elegant solutions.

Core Soul

Dolphins and whales are able to consciously shut down one of their two brain hemispheres, allowing one to remain in resting mode while maintaining the other in full awake mode. In this way, they are never fully unconscious, but still get the rest they need, alternating between the hemispheres as required.

For example, when a dolphin decides to switch off half of its brain to rest, the other half stays alert for possible predators and to remind him to breathe and get its oxygen supply. No other known land mammal is capable of this simultaneous sleep and visually coordinated motion. As the left side of the brain controls the body's right-sided activities and vice versa, the dolphin sleeps with one eye shut, the eye opposite the side of the brain that is resting. Interestingly, humans are anatomically similar in that each of our brain's hemispheres is linked with the eye of the opposite side.

As one dolphin rests, another gently swims under its belly and flips over to face its friend above. This action of conscious effort allows the helping dolphin to switch off the side of its brain that is oppositional to its friend's, meaning he also can enjoy a moment of rest. In this way, the dolphins support each other, acting as one being to stay alert for predators and to facilitate each other's need for sleep.

The first time, I saw this "conscious dolphin sandwich" I was struck mute by the innate intelligence and compassion it revealed. In this example of Nature's brilliance, we are reminded how far we as a human species are removed from the concept of social wholeness and integrity to support the clan as well as the individual, tribe, and society at large. Watching the dolphins' interrelating was the answer to my question about how to birth a healthier civilization. While the tribe acknowledges the individual's needs and desires within it, each tribal member also supports the needs of its next of kin in a perfect cycle of implicit compassion.

The body, with its trillions of interactive cells, and the dolphins, with their advanced communication system, demonstrate the effectiveness of such a superb collective consciousness in its highest form, and outline the best model for an interactive life form. If we want to thrive in a healthy and sustainable way, we have no choice but to adapt and follow this concept of the collective.

Core Soul

In *Spontaneous Evolution*, Bruce Lipton and Steve Bhaerman write: "Like the single-cell organisms that utilized environmental awareness in order to emerge into more complex and efficient organisms, human society must adopt a new paradigm of social and economic relationships. Paradoxically, this new level of cooperative awareness means maximum expression for the individual and maximum benefit for the whole."

Cultivating compassion toward the planet and for our splintered personalities and souls will become an essential feature in the radical change of our conditioned patterns and their existing structures. In this life-sustaining concept, no one is excluded; everyone has the opportunity to participate and contribute to the whole circle of life rather than its individual parts. In this concept of collective consciousness we all benefit. In this communal garden beauty is unchanged and serves as a dance of love between humanity and Nature. If such consciousness can be lived, nothing will be the same. Our relationship to the body and the planet will reflect sacredness and reverence in its very core. We will cherish the divinity deep within the Earth and the divine inherent healing qualities within the body. The body will become a clear reflection of and parallel reality to the possibility of a healthier human civilization.

The New World is meant to bring forth a freedom based on liberation from our small selves in order that we may become an integral part of the larger Self within and of the planet. The New World requires your individual co-creative participation and your eternal dance to manifest itself into form and to be alive. Your conscious efforts are invaluable here; they will not only accelerate the planetary process already in motion, but also deeply contribute to the planetary shift into a wholesome, healthy, and conscious New World. The challenge for us all lies in the level of our individual willingness, devotion, daily practice, and participation in this historic planetary evolution, and in our capacity to implement our individual, eternal, soulful dance as a tool for a completely new way of living.

Core Soul

Our dance comes to an end but only for now, as the dance between old and new is never-ending. Although its nature and intensity may be undefined, this dance gently reminds us of its existence and consistent rhythm. This is the dance of transformation—the transfer of information—moving between opposites until a new place of connectedness takes a foothold.

It is an honor to have danced with you to so many songs, rhythms, and moods, and to allow the full and complete potentiality of such sweet healing to occur. I sincerely hope your dance continues to be an inspiring, vibrant, and joyful experience that becomes your eternal dance and a way of life.

> Another world is not only possible, she is on her way.
> On a quiet day, I can hear her breathing.
>
> —Arudhati Roy

We Have Come To Be Danced

We have come to be danced
Not the pretty dance
Not the pretty pretty, pick me, pick me dance
But the claw our way back into the belly
Of the sacred, sensual animal dance
The unhinged, unplugged, cat is out of its box dance
The holding the precious moment in the palms
Of our hands and feet dance.

We have come to be danced
Not the jiffy booby, shake your booty for him dance
But the wring the sadness from our skin dance
The blow the chip off our shoulder dance.
The slap the apology from our posture dance.

We have come to be danced
Not the monkey see, monkey do dance
One two dance like you
One two three, dance like me dance
but the grave robber, tomb stalker
Tearing scabs and scars open dance
The rub the rhythm raw against our soul dance.

We have come to be danced
Not the nice, invisible, self-conscious shuffle
But the matted hair flying, voodoo mama
Shaman shakin' ancient bones dance

The strip us from our casings, return our wings
Sharpen our claws and tongues dance
The shed dead cells and slip into
The luminous skin of love dance.

We have come to be danced
Not the hold our breath and wallow in the shallow end
of the floor dance
But the meeting of the trinity, the body breath and beat dance
The shout hallelujah from the top of our thighs dance
The mother may I?
Yes you may take 10 giant leaps dance
The olly olly oxen free free free dance
The everyone can come to our heaven dance.

We have come to be danced
Where the kingdoms collide
In the cathedral of flesh
To burn back into the light
To unravel, to play, to fly, to pray
To root in skin sanctuary
We have come to be danced

WE HAVE COME.

—Jewel Mathieson
(poet, dancer, artist, and breast cancer survivor)

Being a self-published independent author,
I appreciate whole-heartedly your book review at Amazon.com

References

The Healing Power of Illness, Thorwald Dethlefsen and Rüdiger Dahlke M.D., Element Books, Inc., 1990.
The Biology of Belief, Bruce H. Lipton, Ph.D. Hay House, Inc., 2008.
The Spontaneous Healing of Belief, Gregg Braden, Hay House, Inc., 2008.
The Other Song, Rajan Sankaran M.D. (Hom), Thomson Press (India) Ltd., 2008.
Vibration Creates Matter, David Icke, YouTube Video, 2009.
Reinventing The Body, Resurrecting the Soul, Deepak Chopra, Random House, Inc., 2011.
Quantum Healing, Deepak Chopra, Bantam Books, 1989.
Yoga and The Quest for the True Self, Stephen Cope, Bantam Books, 2000.
Paracelsus, His Methods of Healing, Douglas Baker, M.R.C.S. L.R.C.P. B.A. F.Z.S. Little Elephant/Douglas Baker, 1986.
Anatomy of the Spirit, Caroline Myss, Ph.D. Three Rivers Press, imprint of Crown Publishing Group, 1996.
"Why Your DNA Isn't Your Destiny," *Time Magazine*, Time Inc., Jan. 2010.
The Pro-Vita Plan, Your Foundation For Optimal Nutrition, Dr. Jack Tips, N.D. Ph.D. Apple-A-Day Press, 1993.
The Healing Triad, Your Liver... Your Lifeline, Dr. Jack Tips, N.D. Ph.D. Apple-A-Day Press, 1986.
Homeopathy, The Principles & Practice of Treatment, Dr. Andrew Lockie and Dr. Nicola Geddes, Dorling Kindersley Book, 1995.
The Secret Teaching of Plants, Stephen Harrod Buhner, Bear & Company, 2004.
Institute of Heart Math, Rollin McCraty, Ph.D. *The HeartMath Solution*, Doc Lew Childre, Howard Martin, Donna Beech, Harper Collins Publication, 1999.
Spiritual Nutrition, Gabriel Cousens, M.D., North Atlantic Books & Essene Vision Books, 2005.

References

Raw Food, Real World, Matthew Kenney and Sarma Melngailis, Regan Books, Imprint of Harper Collins Publishers, 2005.
The Secret Language of Birthdays, Gary Goldschneider & Joost Elffers, Viking Penguin, Division of Penguin Books, 1994.
"The Fires Within," *Time Magazine*, Time Inc., February 2004.
The Benefits of Detoxification, Kirsten Brooks, EnergyGrid Magazine (online magazine), 2007.
The Seat of the Soul, Gary Zukav, Free Press, A Division of Simon & Schuster, Inc., 1989.
The Complete Guide to the Soul, Patrick Harpur, Rider Books, an imprint of Ebury Publishing, 2010.
On the Soul, Aristotle, Digireads.com Publishing, 2006.
Love and the Soul, Robert Sardello, Ph.D., Goldenstone Press, Heaven & Earth Publishing, 2008.
On Soul and Earth, Elena Liotta, Routledge, an imprint of the Taylor & Francis Group, 2009.
Spontaneous Evolution, Bruce H. Lipton, Ph.D. and Steve Bhaerman, Hay House, Inc., 2009.
The Untethered Soul, Michael A. Singer, New Harbinger Publications and Noetic Books, 2007.
Dolphin Connection, Joan Ocean, Dolphin Connection, 1989, 1996.

Websites

Detox Diet-Do It The Right Way, Alternative Medicine, www.altmedicine.about.com
Arizona Center For Advanced Medicine, Scottsdale, www.arizonaadvancedmedicine.com
Fukushima News and Articles: www.naturalnews.com
The Benefits of Detoxifying Your Body: www.livestrong.com
What are Enzymes? www.enzymedica.com
Fermented Food: www.cheeseslave.com/got-bacteria-10-reasons-to-eat-fermented-foods/

References

Babies Microbiomes: www.michaeldomingos.hubpages.com/hub/Babies-Are-Born-Dirty-With-a-Gut-Full-of-Bacteria-New-Research-in-Microbiomes

Normal pH Levels in Humans: www.ehow.com

Amazing Medical Facts of the Body: www.medindia.net

Tonglen Meditation: www.squidoo.com/tonglen

What are Crop Circles? http://science.howstuffworks.com/science-vs-myth/unexplained-phenomena/question735.htm

Women to Women, by Marcelle Pick, OB/GYN: www.womentowomen.com

The Benefits of Detoxification, by Kirsten Brooks: www.energygrid.com/health/2007/07kb-detoxification.html

What is DNA Methylation? www.wisegeek.com/what-is-dna-methylation.htm

How Chronic Cellular Inflammation Ages Skin: blog.perriconemd.com

Article - Man needing transplant stuns doctors when organ mends: www.omaha.com/article/20120923/LIVEWELL01/709239933/1685

Creating Healthy Communities, Healthy Homes, Healthy People: Initiating a Research Agenda on the Built Environment on Public Health
http://ajph.aphapublications.org/doi/abs/10.2105/AJPH.93.9.1446

Creating A Healthy Environment: The Impact of the Built Environment on Public Health, www.sprawlwatch.org/health.pdf

Organic Foods: Health and Environmental Advantages and Disadvantages: www.healthychild.org/blog/comments/how_pesticides_harm_childrens_health_and_brains/#ixzz2AqB7nlOZ

How the environment affects mental health: Michael Rutter, FRCPsych

How hospital environment affect patients and staff: www.guardian.co.uk/sustainable-business/hospital-environment-affect-patients-staff

Meaning of Dolphins: www.whats-your-sign.com/dolphin-meaning-dolphin-symbolism.html

Dolphin Sleep Pattern: http://understanddolphins.tripod.com/dolphinsleeping.html

About the Author

ANGELIKA MARIA KOCH DNM LCH H.N.H.Ir. is a Doctor of Natural Medicine, and the owner of MEDICA NOVA, Practice for Integrated & Educational Medicine. For over three decades in her clinical practice, Angelika Maria Koch has synthesized and applied a unique blend of effective, cutting-edge therapeutic tools in an innovative and holistic approach for her patients' well-being. Utilizing classical homeopathy, iridology, sclerology, systemic herbology, cellular biology, colortherapy, advanced biofeedback, and depth psychology, Angelika Maria Koch passionately continues her deepening exploration of holistic treatments for this complex and unfolding New World. Her extensive international training and education was acquired in England and the United States.

As an adjunct professor of homeopathy, Angelika Maria Koch teaches at the University of New Mexico in Taos and is the author of monthly free newsletters which are published on her website and available via subscription and public social media. For further information and future events, please contact her at: www.medicanova.net.

Angelika Maria Koch, born in Germany, currently resides in Taos, New Mexico. She is the mother of two sons and a proud grandmother.

&

> My aim is to assist you in the communication of your inherent creative intelligence to heal itself and bring forth your pure potentiality. In this way each and every one of us contributes to a better health for humanity.
> —Angelika Maria Koch

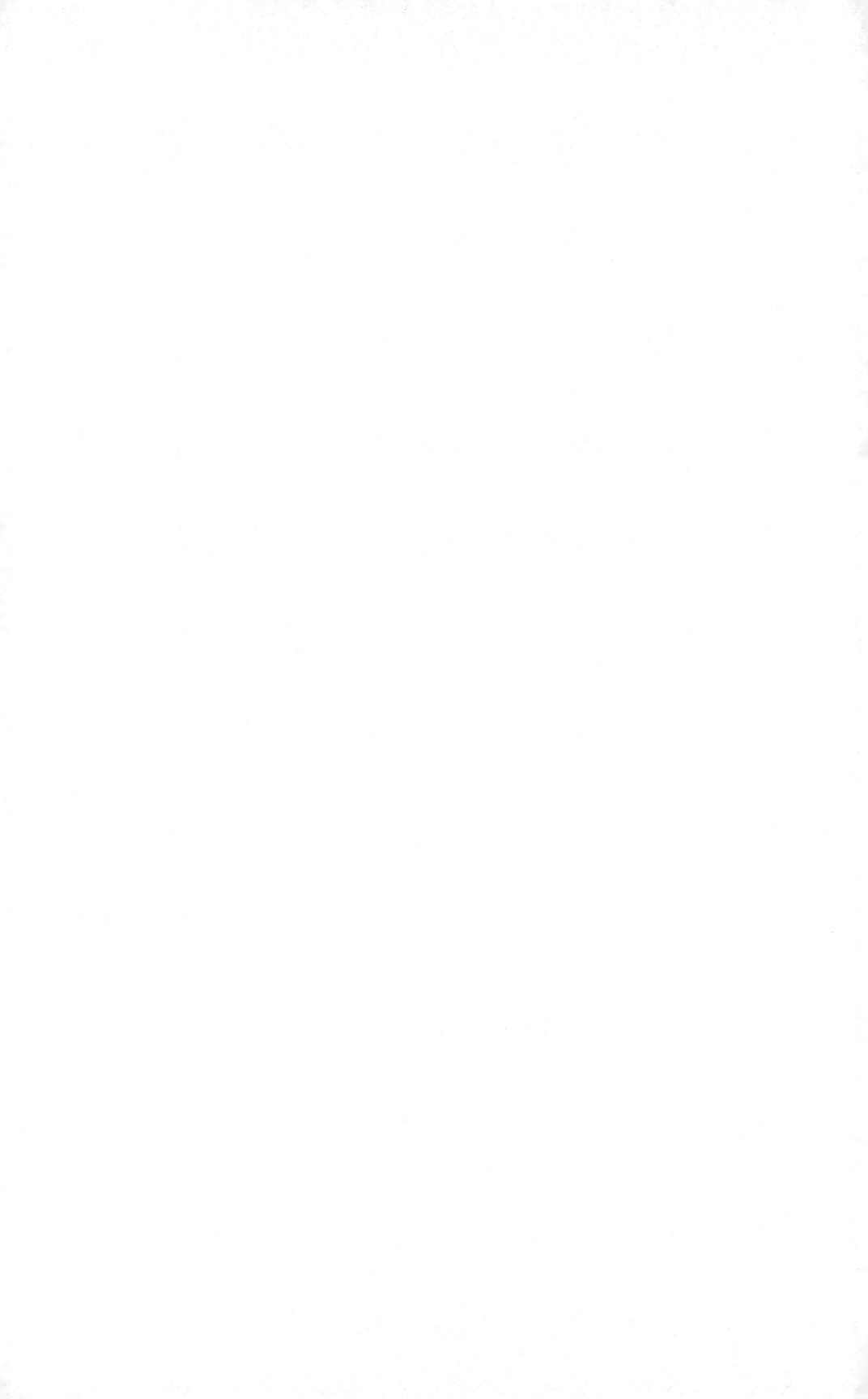

Printed in Great Britain
by Amazon